FAIR MILE HOSPITAL

A VICTORIAN ASYLUM

FAIR MILE HOSPITAL

A VICTORIAN ASYLUM

IAN WHEELER

The History Press

First published 2015

The History Press
The Mill, Brimscombe Port
Stroud, Gloucestershire, GL5 2QG
www.thehistorypress.co.uk

British Library Cataloguing in Publication Data.
A catalogue record for this book is available from the British Library.

ISBN 978 0 7509 5603 1

Typesetting and origination by The History Press
Printed and bound in Malta by Melita Press

CONTENTS

ABOUT THE AUTHOR

....

Born in Oxford in 1950, Ian Wheeler has lived in Cholsey for a total of about forty of the intervening years and has always had strong links with the village. After grammar school in Sidcup, Kent, he pursued a career path which, if not exactly stellar, spoke of a certain versatility, having been involved in banking, sales, purchasing, scientific research, business computing, health and safety, quality assurance and piloting trains and white vans at frightening speeds. He now edits medical and scientific research papers for major international publishers and blesses his former English teachers.

When not working, Ian is a keen performing folk musician, choral singer, model maker, aviation buff and morris dancer. It's a dirty job but someone has to do it.

INTRODUCTION

··

> There they stand, isolated, majestic, imperious, brooded over by the gigantic water-tower and chimney combined, rising unmistakable and daunting out of the countryside – the asylums which our forefathers built with such immense solidity to express the notions of their day.

Enoch Powell, 'The Water Tower Speech', 1961

Despite its many achievements, Victorian society was as imperfect as most and nowadays we tend to call to mind aspects that were unjust and unthinkable by today's 'enlightened' standards. Contrasting with great affluence in some quarters, we learn of devastating poverty, deprivation, the dreaded workhouse, disease and rigid social demarcation: images of Bethlem Hospital ('Bedlam') are seldom far from the mind when the subject of mental illness is mentioned.

Yet by the time Queen Victoria was on the throne, there was a fashion for social responsibility and philanthropy and those in authority were quite capable of recognising that mental illness was a condition that deserved sympathetic attention. Society still preferred not to let insanity walk the streets and, in the

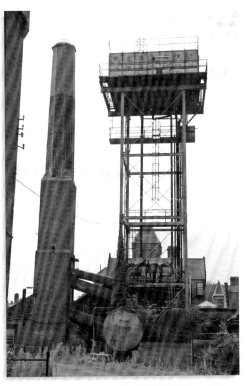

The 1930s water tower dwarfs Fair Mile in this 2010 view. (Bill Nicholls)

absence of what we nowadays recognise as psychiatric therapy, it was thought better to confine the sufferers for the greater good. Although care of the mentally unwell represented a drain on the public purse, there was clearly a strong desire to protect the vulnerable and to find the means of returning them to a normal life. The very word 'asylum', for so long associated with confinement and inner torment, still means *a place of safety*.

The institution that came to be known as Fair Mile Hospital was the product of responsible legislation, improving awareness of the plight of the mentally ill, dedication and hard-won experience. As such it mirrors the achievements of many similar establishments across the counties of the United Kingdom, which opened their doors at about the same time and in similar circumstances. Although smaller than most, it also resembled many of these in physical form, methods of operation, conditions of work and care, and the inevitable challenges of progress and national crisis. Its impact on patients, staff and the unassuming village of Cholsey was profound and, although closed in 2003, it has left a huge legacy in terms of skills, community relations and fond memories. By the mid-twentieth century, scarcely a family in Cholsey was without some sort of connection with Fair Mile. It served as a social hub (notably in the dark days of the Second World War), entered floats in local carnivals and welcomed visitors to its regular garden fêtes. Although standing apart, Fair Mile was embraced by its host village.

The hospital suffered tragedy at times, but also laughter and gaiety. Many amusing and revealing anecdotes still burn brightly in the memories of former staff and their families. Although these are not all suitable for publication, since they might appear to mock the psychologically disadvantaged, I feel it would be foolish not to

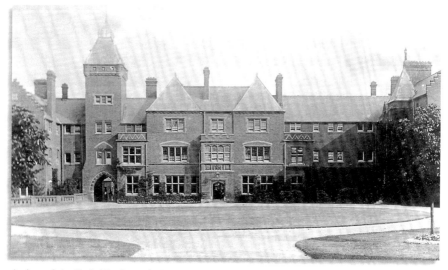

A view of the Berkshire Lunatic Asylum from about 1900. The ornate top to the water tower is fictional and a crude attempt at retouching. (Spackman collection)

confront the issues that they raise by relating some of them impartially. Similarly, some indecorous subjects were bound to arise from such a setting and, since we seeking to understand the hospital, they have been faced head-on.

In *Fair Mile Hospital: A Victorian Asylum* I hope to present a fair portrait of an establishment which, in serving principally the counties of Berkshire and Oxfordshire, exercised a huge influence on Cholsey and its surrounding area, not to mention the thousands of staff and patients who passed through its gates. Whilst accuracy has been my constant aim, some information has required inter-pretation and even some official records appear to contradict each other. I ask forgiveness for any factual errors.

My qualification for compiling this work is largely one of deep interest and family connections. I represent the fourth and last generation of my family to have worked at Fair Mile – fleeting though my association was. The hospital was also my first home for a few months in 1950; I take a small, perverse pleasure in this fact and I hope that content drawn from my family's links with Fair Mile will be suitably entertaining.

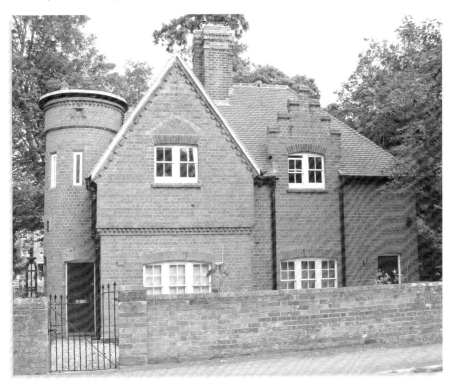

The front Lodge in 2014. From 1927 Leslie Talbot, recently appointed as Hall Porter, lived here with his new wife Lilian and raised two children. The author – the Talbots' newly arrived first grandchild – joined his parents in sharing the cottage for a few months in 1950. Incredibly, the turret houses a bedroom. (Author's collection)

Readers will notice that much of the information offered refers to the period prior to the advent of the National Health Service. This is because records from later than 1948 are relatively sparse. All the records that survived to the hospital's closure were acquired and catalogued by the Berkshire Record Office (BRO) and some classes of information are currently closed to public examination out of consideration for former patients' privacy. If this leads to uncomfortable gaps in this account, I share your disappointment.

It is important to acknowledge the key role of Mr Tony Spackman, Mental Health Service Manager at Fair Mile in its final years, who made available to me a collection of archive photographs, many appearing herein, that inspired the research for this project.

The words asylum and hospital, as well as Fair Mile and other official appellations, are used interchangeably to reflect the changes of name imposed on the establishment over the years, and every effort has been made to use the most appropriate term for the period under discussion. The same caveat applies to the whereabouts of the asylum, variously recorded as Moulsford, Wallingford and Cholsey. Be in no doubt, however, that the true location has always been Cholsey.

This project was made possible by the foresight and generosity of people who cared for Fair Mile and its patients, and who have kindly added their memories to those of my family. It is to all of these that I dedicate this book.

Ian Wheeler, 2015

1

ORIGINS AND
FOUNDATION

Madness, lunacy, insanity, derangement, mental imbalance, psychosis. Whatever term chosen, the problem is essentially the same: a person has in some way lost the ability to think as a normal member of a society, family, social group or perhaps workforce, may be at personal risk and could represent a danger to others. The cause may be rooted in personal tragedy, physical illness, loss, conflict, deprivation or discrimination. Whilst this book cannot begin to explain mental illness or the invaluable work over many decades of researchers, sociologists, carers and chemists to bring relief, it is at least clear that, during the 1800s, mentally ill people were considered deserving of assistance.

The story of Fair Mile Hospital begins with the passing of the Lunacy Act of 1845 and the foundation of the Lunacy Commission under the noted social reformer, Lord Shaftesbury. The Act strengthened hitherto inadequate provisions for the so-called 'pauper lunatics' who, under the County Asylums Act of 1808, at least enjoyed the official status of 'patients'. Somewhat paradoxically, the 1845 Act removed patients' legal right to challenge their detention through the courts but, alongside the County Asylums Act of 1845, it did make them the responsibility of the counties instead of relying on their families, the parishes – possibly through recourse to the workhouse – or the prisons. All the same, given the cost of caring for and treating the mentally unwell, admission to an asylum was to be far from a foregone conclusion.

In 1845, Wallingford, Cholsey, Moulsford and other communities in what was to be Fair Mile's catchment area stood firmly in the county of Berkshire[1], which had no mental care facilities of its own. Instead, under an 1847 agreement or 'union' with the Berkshire Court of Quarter Sessions, Littlemore Asylum, near Oxford – itself founded only in 1846 – shouldered this burden. The boroughs of Abingdon and Windsor are recorded as separate parties to this union, with Reading joining a little later; all eventually withdrew from the Littlemore agreement and subscribed to Berkshire's arrangements as they developed. Meanwhile, the provision of asylum facilities became compulsory in 1853.

Unfortunately – at least partly due to the primitive therapies available to medical science at the time – Littlemore's patient population burgeoned until, in 1867, it was abundantly clear that the Royal County would have to create its own facility. This precipitated a fresh union between the Berkshire Court of Quarter Sessions and the boroughs of Reading and Newbury, under which a new asylum would be built. Situated more or less equidistant from the villages of Moulsford and Cholsey – though very much in the ancient parish of Cholsey – it was to be known as the Moulsford Asylum. If the reader should become confused over the asylum's name and whereabouts, some clarification is offered in Chapter 2.

In 1867, a Committee of Visitors, assembled under the auspices of the Berkshire Court of Quarter Sessions, appointed Charles Henry Howell, FRIBA, of Lancaster Place, London, as the asylum's architect. At the age of 43 he was already holding the august position of Consulting Architect to the Commissioners in Lunacy. Howell was responsible for a number of comparable asylums including Brookwood (opening in 1868), Beverley (1871), Cane Hill (1883) and Middlesbrough (1898). The appointed building contractors were Mansfield, Price & Co. of London.

The asylum's site, purchased from the locally prominent Hedges family (at the time, owners of Wallingford Castle), occupied 67 acres in a roughly rectangular plot between the Reading turnpike (now the A329) and the River Thames.[2] Its south-western boundary was the lane[3] linking Cholsey to the Little Stoke ferry and, to the east, the long river frontage incorporated water meadows to the north and south. Its position and orientation were considered very favourable – not least for the wellbeing of the patients – enjoying good air and pleasant views.

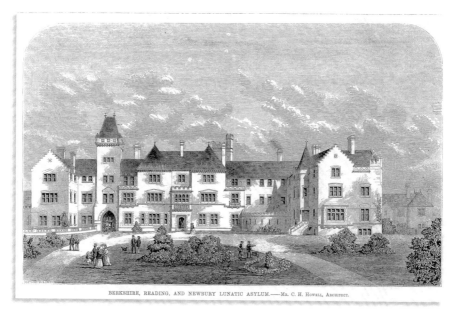

BERKSHIRE, READING, AND NEWBURY LUNATIC ASYLUM.——Mr. C. H. Howell, Architect.

This engraving appeared in *The Builder* in 1869. (Spackman collection)

With the turnpike road passing its front gate, the asylum had good communications with Wallingford, 2 miles distant. However, given the troubles that still affected road travel in poor weather, the proximity of Moulsford railway station was highly advantageous as it afforded easy travel to London and Bristol and a branch line service to Wallingford.

Conceived – like other asylums of the day – as an almost self-sufficient community, Howell's creation would initially accommodate 133 male and 152 female patients – a total of 285, with plans for growth to 500. With associated staff they would dwell in an imposing, three-storeyed red-and-blue-brick pile with a front range boasting stone mullions, 'crow step' gables and a slate-covered roofline, which spoke broadly of Victorian ambition and pride.[4] Away from public view, the architecture was rather more prosaic, although still on a grand scale. Much care was put into the layout being fit for purpose, one important feature being that newly arrived and 'acute' cases were accommodated away from busy areas and thoroughfares.

The plan on page 14 shows the three major phases of the asylum's development up to 1904 and identifies Male and Female wards, kitchen with attendant scullery and pantry, a dining hall, committee room, offices, an extensive laundry, workshops for boot makers, tailors, mattress stuffing and hair picking – not forgetting a substantial residence for the Superintendent who, from his front windows, was able to survey the Oval, the turning circle for carriages that served the asylum's dignified front entrance. The wards were numbered Male 1, 2, 3 and Female 1, 2, 3, etc., not taking names until 1959. Staff spoke of 'Male twos', 'Female eights' and so forth for years afterwards.

The internal arrangements altered with the growth of the asylum and Male and Female wards were originally situated to both north (left) and south (right) of the main entrance. Those to the north were more secure, having smaller windows and being equipped with padded rooms, while those to the south housed new admissions and convalescents and had better access to the grounds. But, by 1904, each sex was firmly confined to its own half of the premises as shown, and this remained the accepted pattern.

Howell's scheme was comprehensive. A mixed farm, orchard and kitchen gardens were to be created to both help feed the asylum's occupants and provide gainful activity for the patients. A gas works and 'gasometer' (properly known as a gas holder) were installed on the northern boundary to serve the lighting arrangements and 'dry furnaces' heated the wards via hot air ducts (central heating arrived later, as explained in Chapter 3). There were to be extensive pleasure grounds with wooded margins, laid out by notable landscape designer Robert Marnock and planted with a veritable arboretum of species[5] by a Mr Joseph Harding, nurseryman, of nearby Winterbrook. There would also be a spring to provide sweet drinking water and a chapel to cater for the spiritual needs of all.

Construction began in March 1868 and a number of outlying cottages went up at an early stage, housing workmen before passing to the key employees as

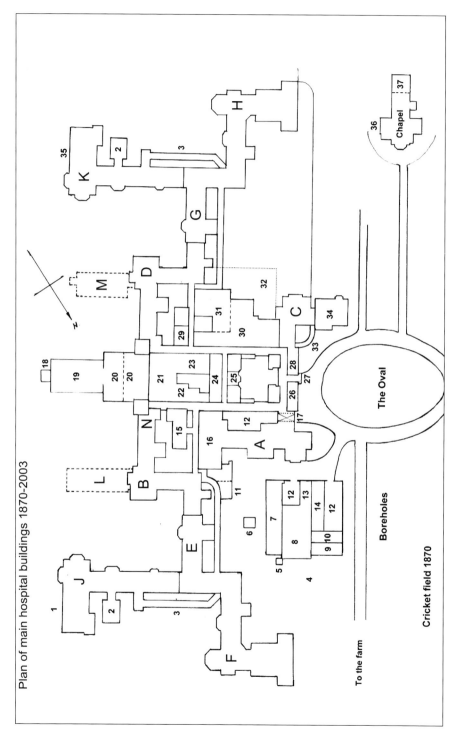

Plan of main hospital buildings 1870–2003

(Author)

Following the phases of building, the wards were numbered from 1 to 9 on each side. The change to ward names in 1959 used an alphabetical sequence that echoed the original numbering but no explanation can be found as to why Female 8 became Ipsden, while Female 9 was Henley.

Phase	Key	Ground floor	First floor	Second floor
1870 Original	A	Male 1 (Aldworth)		
	B	Male 2 (Blewbury)	Male 3 (Compton)	
	C	Female 1 (Aldermaston)		
	D	Female 2 (Basildon)	Female 3 (Caversham)	
1881 Howell's extensions	E	Male 4 (Drayton; later Ridgeway)	Male 5 (Easthampstead; later Ridgeway)	
	F	Male 6 (Frilsham)	Male 7 (Grazeley)	Male Top 7 (Grazeley)
	G	Female 4 (Didcot)	Female 5 (Englefield)	
	H	Female 6 (Faringdon)	Female 7 (Goring)	Female Top 7 (Goring)
1902 Hine's extensions	J	Male 8 (Hermitage)	Male 9 (Ilsley)	
	K	Female 8 (Ipsden)	Female 9 (Henley)	
c.1958	L	Blewbury dormitory extension (male)	Compton dormitory extension (male)	
	M	Basildon dormitory extension (female)	Caversham dormitory extension (female)	
Post-1959	N			Yattendon (mixed)

1	Verandah from c.1929 (position of)		19	Recreation Hall 1881
2	Sanitary annexe		20	Dining hall (extended 1881)
3	External corridor (ground floor only; four examples)		21	Kitchen
			22	Scullery and vegetable store
4	Water tower c.1935 (site of)		23	Meat store and pantry
5	Boiler house chimney		24	General Stores
6	Fire pump house (later superseded)		25	Mess room, Surgery and Committee room (first floor added 1902)
7	Battery and engine room, workshop and stoker's bedroom		26	Committee Room
8	Boiler house 1900 (old boiler house adjacent)		27	Main entrance
			28	Office
9	Mortuary		29	Female officers' mess and recreation room
10	Shed		30	Laundry 1870–1960
11	Bakery extension 1900		31	Laundry extension c.1900
12	Yard		32	New kitchen 1960–2003 (dotted outline)
13	Coal store		33	Curved corridor
14	Establishment workshops		34	Medical Superintendent's residence 1870–1931
15	Male officers' mess and recreation room			
16	Workshops for bootmakers, mattresses and hair picking		35	Verandah from 1927 (position of)
			36	Transepts added 1881
17	Water tower		37	Chapel extension c.1900
18	Projection room c.1939			

THE OVAL

The Oval was sacrosanct and had its own traditions. Its grassed centre was not to be walked upon, on pain of disciplinary action, and was jealously tended and mown using a horse-drawn mower operated by a 'working' patient: the luckless pony was outfitted with overshoes that spread its weight, avoiding damage to the turf.

A celebrated tradition was that male staff approaching or leaving the main entrance door were required to walk on the path to the north of the Oval, while female staff passed by the south side.

'emoluments' befitting their positions. Still occupied, these were two pairs of cottages on the Reading Road boundary and a terrace just to the south-west of the site.

The Moulsford Asylum opened its doors on 30 September 1870 and an extract from the first report of the Committee of Visitors (covering the period 30 September 1870 to 31 December 1871) recalls that, discounting some small change, expenditure had amounted to £8,317 for the site, £46,299 for construction and around £3,500 for 'the gas works and fittings, the pumps and steam engine and pipes, and the auxiliary heating apparatus'. A further £9,116 had to be invested in 'fittings, furniture, clothing, stocking of farm, road-making, ground levelling'.

This investment was placed under the guiding hand of Dr Robert Bryce Gilland, Medical Superintendent, who supervised the first arrivals from Littlemore Asylum and set about creating the necessary caring environment. Gilland was a 32-year-old bachelor who had previously been Assistant Medical Superintendent at both the Glasgow Royal Asylum at Gartnavel and the Essex County Lunatic Asylum near Brentwood. His experience would be the bedrock that supported him through seventeen trying years at Moulsford.

The first available superintendent's monthly report is dated 20 January 1871 and records the death of a female patient from pneumonia, the arrival of a new hall porter, the expeditious vaccination of 'patients and servants' (although it is not stated for which disease), the arrival of a number of patients from Camberwell[6] and a request from Littlemore that Gilland take 'a few of' (their) worst female patients'. In addition to this, patient numbers – including details of arrivals, discharges and deaths – were recorded in a table pre-printed into the ledger. It seems that the ink was hardly dry on this page before the incoming hall porter had second thoughts and another had to be found. Each report of this kind was examined by the Committee of Visitors and countersigned.

The May report detailed Gilland's delight at the success of the vaccination programme but a marked increase in patient numbers and dismay at destructive female admissions 'of the worst class', who exhibited lamentably poor personal hygiene – probably better left to the imagination. Sadly, there was also scandal among the attendants, with mention of 'probable concealment of birth and infanticide'.

By 16 June, Gilland was appealing to the Committee of Visitors to avoid placing elderly, incurable cases in his charge, claiming that it was unfair when the asylum 'is so suited to the recovery of younger patients'. This sounds unsympathetic but numerous subsequent entries show that some new arrivals, often very elderly, arrived from the workhouses in a wretched condition and terminally ill, their troublesome symptoms owing much to the poor standards of care they had received from the parish. Meanwhile, amid 'much difficulty in finding suitable attendants', Gilland was striving to create a beneficial and positive environment by purchasing equipment for outdoor games, engravings to enhance the interior decor and, that same month, engaging 'a trio of Italian strolling musicians who, with harp and violins, played in an exquisite manner' to the evident enjoyment of those patients well enough to attend.

Another major item of concern, always reported in tones of regret, was the deaths of patients. The commonest causes during the first eighteen months of operation were exhaustion, sometimes associated with melancholy; phthisis (nowadays known as pulmonary tuberculosis or TB); diarrhoea (with one mention of dysentery); apoplexy (stroke); erysipelas (a streptococcal infection) and 'general paralysis of the insane', which is brain damage associated with late-stage syphilis. Had Gilland had access to modern anti-depressive drugs and antibiotics, his unenviable position as custodian of these poor cases would have been much easier. As it was, he was frequently at pains to defend the best available efforts, especially when a death occurred during one of his very rare leaves of absence.

An item of note in the 1871 journals is the employment of male patients in the filling of gravel pits dug during the asylum's construction, improving the turnpike road and creating 'a store of dry earth for the closets'. Although water closets were certainly in place, the modern plumbing might have been less than ubiquitous.

Based on samples from these enlightening reports, it is clear that Superintendent Gilland's daily concerns revolved around patient capacity, continuing difficulty in recruiting reliable personnel, efforts to fill new staff positions, such as Housekeeper, Shoemaker and Tailor, the repair of defective workmanship in the buildings and the quality and quantity of the foodstuffs provided to sustain the patients. Indeed his estimable successors seldom fared better for a century thereafter.

All of these aspects of the asylum's day-to-day operation, and more, are examined in the following chapters.

2

GOVERNANCE AND MANAGEMENT

....

Names Used by Fair Mile Hospital

1870–97	The Moulsford Asylum
1897–*c.*1915	The Berkshire Lunatic Asylum, although a set of printed regulations dated 1904 clearly uses 'The Berkshire Asylum, Wallingford'. The front cover of Volume 9 of the Visitors' Minute Book (commencing 1908) is boldly gilt-embossed with 'Berkshire Pauper Lunatic Asylum' and the style 'Berks County Asylum' has been found here and there. There are yet more variations, including Berkshire County Lunatic Asylum, which is highly convincing as it follows the standard pattern across the country.
*c.*1915–1948	The Berkshire Mental Hospital (BMH). The date remains uncertain and could be as late as 1920. Rather annoyingly, the 1927 update of the Staff Regulations still states 'at Wallingford'. The Commissioners to the Board of Control used 'Berkshire Mental Hospital' up to 1939 but inserted 'County' thereafter. This detail clearly didn't reach everyone's attention.
1948–2010	Fair Mile Hospital. Mercifully, no dissention has yet been uncovered, apart from a tendency to write 'Fairmile'. Fair Mile is taken from a broad, straight and very ancient drove road in the nearby Berkshire Downs, connecting with The Ridgeway.
From 2010	With the commencement of redevelopment for housing, the new-build areas of the site took the name Cholsey Meadows, to the puzzlement of local residents. The listed Victorian buildings, however, underwent their renaissance as Fair Mile, with some of the ward names being retained.

The Commissioners in Lunacy were a body of worthies established under the provisions of the Lunacy Act of 1845. Succeeding the Metropolitan Commissioners in Lunacy, they had influence outside the London area, overseeing the many county asylums for 'pauper lunatics' that were set up as a consequence of the Act. From 1914, following the 1913 Mental Deficiency Act, the Commissioners acted under the aegis of the Board of Control for Lunacy and Mental Deficiency, which superseded the Lunacy Commission and had additional responsibility for mental defectives. The Board of Control originally reported to the Home Office but fell under the Ministry of Health from 1919 as a result of fresh legislation. These changes apart, the way the asylum was regulated appears to have remained largely unaltered.

Responsibility for establishing and running the asylums fell to the county authorities; in Berkshire's case, this devolved to the magistrates via the Berkshire Court of Quarter Sessions, which set up a 'union' between the County of Berkshire and the boroughs of Reading and Newbury (sometimes referred to as 'the Bodies in Union'). The court also appointed a Committee of Visitors, some of them clearly Justices of the Peace, charged with ensuring the sound management, governance and financial control of the asylums. Committee members included 'visitors' from the boroughs subscribing to the union which, in 1896, welcomed the Borough of New Windsor, followed in 1898 by Henley, which embraced Caversham. The Royal Borough of Windsor joined in 1908. Meanwhile, the Lunacy Act of 1890 transferred responsibility from the courts to the county councils.

Arrangements were made to transport the numerous Visitors to and from their monthly meetings at Moulsford and they were afforded the services of a clerk: Mr John Thornhill Morland MA was Clerk to the Visitors from 1870 until at least 1909.

Until 1892, Moulsford's railway station stood an easy walk from the asylum's gates, on Brunel's Great Western line from London to Bristol. This was a convenient means of bringing some of the Visitors to meetings. In January 1909, although the station had necessarily been relocated half a mile further west (and renamed Cholsey and Moulsford), Morland was instructed to write to the Great Western Railway requesting a special train on meeting days for the convenience of the Committee. Although the running of special services was in those days a means by which any self-respecting railway could solicit the approval of the Great and the Good, the GWR's reply very respectfully turned them down flat.

The superintendent, his senior officers and the chaplain were bound by the Committee's decisions and required to keep journals of the execution of their duties. This did not mean that the superintendent was without influence; he was charged with applying his professional judgement to prevailing circumstances but many measures – notably those involving expenditure – had to be ratified by the Visitors with a degree of formality that might nowadays be summed up as 'starchy'.

MEDICAL SUPERINTENDENTS 1870–1965

1870–86   Dr Robert Bryce Gilland, the first medical superintendent, was clearly passionate about his responsibilities. Formerly Assistant Medical Officer at the Essex County Asylum, Warley, Essex, he presided at Moulsford until 1886, rarely taking holiday and quitting his duties only when ill health left him no alternative. He reported in July that year that he was in need of a rest and requested leave of absence – simultaneously expressing regret that no locum tenens[7] had yet been found to cover his absence. Dr James Murdoch was by this time his Assistant Medical Officer and Gilland generously suggested that 'Dr Murdoch, by himself, would be quite able to take charge of the asylum'. This was duly ratified and on 20 August 1886, Gilland dutifully recorded his thanks to the Committee for both his leave and their approval of Dr Murdoch as stand-in.

Dr Gilland took leave of the Moulsford Asylum that October and never returned. He died on 8 March 1887, having effectively worked himself to death at the age of 49.

1886–87   Dr John Barron, also Assistant Medical Officer, actually took over on Gilland's departure instead of Dr Murdoch and served until a new superintendent was appointed.

1887–92   Dr Joel Harrington Douty, who qualified to practice medicine in 1881 and, at 29 years of age, was the youngest superintendent who served at the asylum, arrived with his wife and young son. He was evidently progressive and innovative, for he promptly prepared a long list of items deserving the attention of the Committee of Visitors, requesting their guidance in respect of irrigation of land, beer money for attendants (50*s* male and 40*s* female per annum were granted), mowing equipment, the Queen's Jubilee, a fire brigade, the purchase of a large 'Cyclostyle'[8] for cheaply printing dietary tables 'in house' and 'Repair of the electric tell-tale apparatus'.[9]

His reports show concern over morale, reward where merited and the poverty of some patients' families, who would care for their relatives if they had the means. He recommended 'a small weekly allowance' from the asylum until they could find employment.

Douty unfortunately died after a short illness at the age of 34, only five years after his arrival. His death certificate was signed by his deputy, Dr Hugh Attwood Beaver, who is understood to have run away to Canada with Douty's young widow shortly afterwards. Superintendent Douty is buried in Cholsey churchyard, close to a number of his patients.

1892–1917   Dr James William Aitken Murdoch. A determined and industrious Scot, Dr Murdoch's reputation as a good doctor endured long after his unfortunate death, late in 1917, following an operation for appendicitis. He joined as Assistant Medical Officer in 1881 and in April 1892, after six years' service as Deputy Superintendent, was considered for Medical Superintendent at the Kent County Asylum, Chartham. He succeeded the unfortunate Dr Douty that same year and was outspoken in his criticism of unsuitable cases being foisted on his undertaking. Dr Murdoch was also conservative and suspicious of change in a field of endeavour where progress was necessary and unavoidable; it was several years before he could be persuaded to attend conferences on the advancement of psychiatric medicine. He is buried in Cholsey churchyard.

1918–20   Dr Edwin Lindsay Dunn. Born in Waterside, Ireland, Dunn became Assistant Medical Officer and Deputy Superintendent at the Berkshire Lunatic Asylum in 1894, succeeding Dr Murdoch at the start of 1918. He was highly intelligent, well informed and an active researcher in his field, with a keen sense of humour that endeared him to staff and patients alike. He sadly died in service in 1920 after a painful illness lasting several weeks. His gravestone can still be found in Cholsey churchyard.

1920–38   Dr Walter Woolfe Read. Born in 1880, Dr Read arrived from Littlemore as Assistant Medical Officer in January 1919, soon becoming Acting Medical Superintendent. Promotion was thrust upon him with the demise of Dr Dunn in 1920 and he was the first superintendent fortunate enough to hand over the title whilst still breathing – which feat he achieved in March 1938. Wry humour apart, the responsibilities of the position were clearly very stressful.

1938–44   Dr Hugh Astley Cooper. Formerly Deputy Medical Superintendent at Hampshire County Mental Hospital at Knowle, Cooper assumed his position on 1 April 1938 and was almost certainly a descendent of Sir Astley Paston Cooper, an eminent surgeon of the nineteenth century. Little has come to light to characterise his tenure and he was dismissed in 1944[10]. He joined the army in a medical capacity, being promoted to lieutenant on 28 October 1944 and acquitting himself well.

1944–*c.*1965 Dr William Ogden was Assistant Medical Officer in 1942 and became Superintendent on the departure of Hugh Astley Cooper in September 1944. He was immediately under heavy pressure to remedy many deficiencies described in these pages. Dr Ogden was competent, popular and much respected by his staff. He was the last superintendent under that title. Although the National Archives quote 1949 as the end of his tenure, he was still in post in the 1960s, retiring in about 1965.

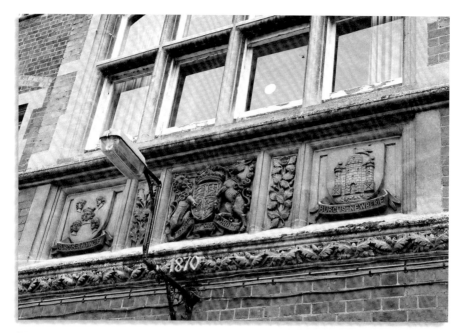

Heraldry over the asylum's front door. Reading's coat of arms, on the left, was changed in 1953 and Newbury's in 1948. (Bill Nicholls)

As mentioned in Chapter 1, the Union's initial strategy had been to pay for beds at Littlemore Asylum (in Oxfordshire) but time brought the need for Berkshire's own hospital. This brings us back to Moulsford, where the Committee appointed agents, architects and builders, selected candidates for the senior staff positions and held the purse strings for all but the most routine expenditure. The Medical Superintendent was supported by various officers but the Clerk of Works[11] may have been among the busiest of these.

The minute books kept by the Clerk to the Committee of Visitors are, alas, incomplete. The earliest survivor commences in 1908 and in December of that year the Committee was made up of Mr P. Wroughton, Chairman; Mr Harris; Mr Barningham; Major Turner; Mr Dockar Drysdale; Mr Isaac; Mr Petrocokino; Lord George Pratt; Dr Stewart Abram; Col Ricardo (Visitor for Berkshire); Mr Martin (Visitor for Reading); Mr Parfitt (ditto); Mr Long (Visitor for Newbury) and Alderman Edward Bampfylde (Visitor for Windsor).

A number of these gentlemen still served in 1912. A list of those present, taken at random, shows Mr J.W. Martin, Vice-Chairman, presiding; Lord George Pratt; Major C. Turner; Mr A.K. Loyd, KC; Col Ricardo; Mr J. Cobb; Mr E.A. Hanley; Mr H. Bate; Mr A. Petrocokino[12]; Mr H. Goddard (Visitor for Berkshire); Dr Stewart Abram (Visitor for Reading); Mr J. Elliott (ditto) and Sir William Shipley (Visitor for Windsor). The earliest credible date for the upper photograph on page 23 is 1912 and it is likely that at least several of those depicted appear in this list.

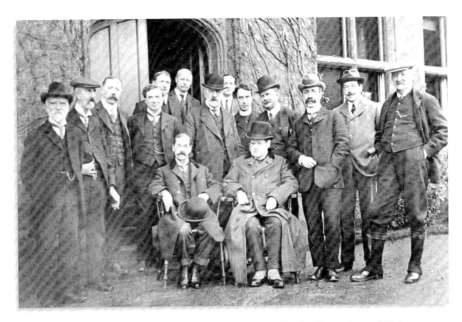

Dr James William Aitken Murdoch (in spats) surrounded by the Committee of Visitors between 1912 and 1917. Mr Moses Nicholls, Clerk and Steward, stands framed by the door. A young Revd Philip Raynor is in clerical collar. Seated next to Dr Murdoch may be Mr J.W. Martin, Chairman of the Committee. (Spackman collection)

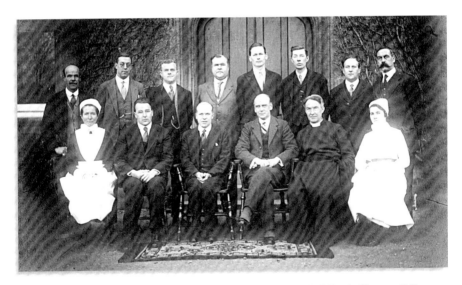

Senior officers in about 1930. Standing, from left: unknown; J.R.F. Davis, Finance Officer; unknown; Avery Nicholls, Steward; Alan Barnard, Assistant Clerk; Mr Walton, Head Male Attendant; Jack Croxford, Deputy Head Male Attendant; Bill Southby, Clerk of Works. Seated, from left: Matron Mary Ratcliffe; unknown; Dr Sidney Holder; Dr Woolfe Read, Medical Superintendent; Revd Philip Raynor, Chaplain; Grace Kirk, Deputy Head Female Nurse. (Spackman collection)

The typical monthly agenda for the Committee of Visitors would be:

- Read the previous meetings' minutes
- Examination of various accounts, bankers' pass books
- Examination of medical superintendent's report
- Read the chaplain's journal
- Review recommendations for discharge of convalescent patients
- Consider any matters of moment, such as planned repairs, improvements, out-of-course expenditure
- Appointments, resignations, etc.
- Read the visitors' book
- Sign cheques
- Tour the hospital to view as many patients as practicable

The Bodies in Union, namely Berkshire, Reading, Newbury and later Windsor, each had an allocation of beds and the costs associated with caring for their residents were charged back to them at a standard rate, calculated for and periodically reviewed by the Committee of Visitors. In May 1887, the ordinary rate for upkeep of patients was 14*s* per week. Rather surprisingly, the rate had dropped to 9*s* 0½*d* by December 1909 and was held at this level for some time. Private patients, when accepted, were charged at a slightly higher rate. A full account would be dull but by 1947 the ordinary rate had risen to 37*s* 4*d*, while private patients were paying 44*s* 4*d*.

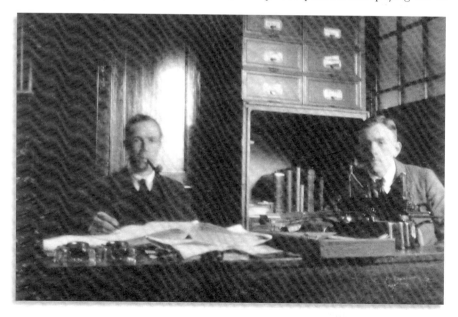

Mr Buffham (with pipe) and Assistant Clerk Jack Lambert in about 1925. (Vera Wheeler)

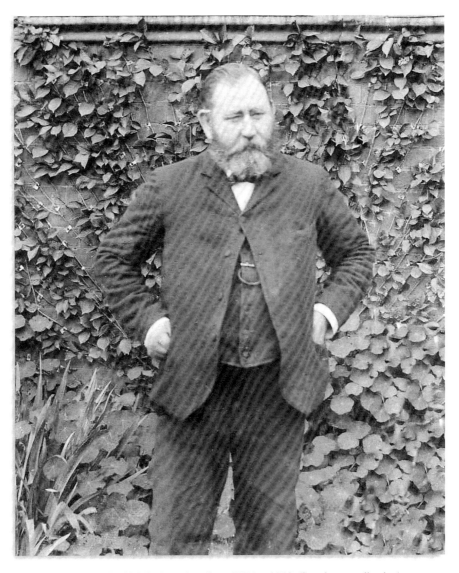

Mr Alfred Lockie, Head Male Attendant from 1874 to 1903. (Spackman collection)

In the day-to-day operation of the asylum, the medical superintendent was supported by medical and administrative officers, nursing staff – known as 'attendants' – and artisan staff. Office accommodation and a meeting room were situated in the front range of the asylum.

The nursing staff acted under the direction of the superintendent or his assistant medical officer(s), with head male and female attendants in charge of exclusively male attendants for the Male side and female attendants for the Female side. Mixed-sex nursing did not emerge until the 1960s.

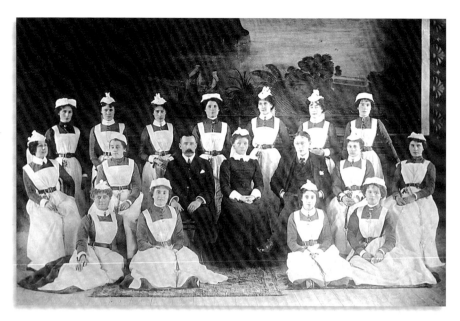

Female attendants, possibly *c.*1910, in which case the lady in black may be either Miss Browne or Miss Jones, Housekeeper. The gentlemen are probably the assistant medical officers of the time. (Spackman collection)

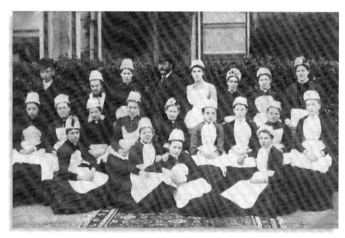

Domestic staff in about 1895. The gentleman, centre, may be Clerk and Steward Moses Nicholls, and the lady to his right may be the Housekeeper, possibly Mrs Horton. Alice Wells is front, second from left. (Spackman collection)

A sizeable contingent of domestic staff, mostly female, was supervised by the housekeeper, with perhaps some influence from the Steward, which may explain the presence of a gentleman in the picture above. Some of the women acted as maids to the doctors but we can be reasonably sure that the majority had general household duties, or else worked in the kitchen, scullery, laundry and needlework room.

Just one example of the asylum's staff establishment shows that 'outsourcing' was far from the Victorian mind. Whilst space prevents an account of everyone on the following list from 1896–97, a few names are offered from research:

- Medical Superintendent Dr James William Aitken Murdoch
- Second Assistant Medical Officer Dr Thomas Leonard Johnston
- Chaplain, Revd F.T. Stewart-Dyer
- Clerk to Visitors, Mr J.T. Morland
- Steward and Clerk of the asylum, Mr Moses Nicholls
- Housekeeper, Miss Browne
- Head Male Attendant, Mr Alfred Lockie
- Head Female Attendant, Miss Edith M. Bearpark
- Superintendent's clerk and organist
- Stores Assistant
- Foreman of Works
- Engineer
- Farm Bailiff, Mr Christian Henry Ellis Carter
- Gatekeeper
- Gardener
- Baker
- Carpenter
- Two painters
- Bricklayer
- Gasman, possibly Mr Hill
- Two stokers, including Mr Ernest J. Brignall
- Shoemaker Attendant, possibly Mr Robert Townley
- Tailor Attendant
- 24 Male Attendants including Mr Frederick Pilgrim and Mr Jack Woolley
- 28 Female Attendants
- 10 indoor servants and laundrymaids, including Miss Alice Wells
- Hall Porter
- Eight farm and garden servants

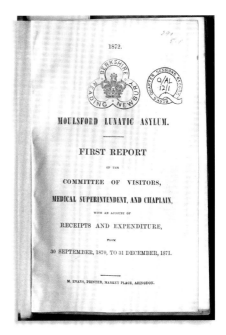

Hardback books were prepared, containing summarised annual reports. These might cover several years per volume and do much to explain the monthly notes found in the Visitors' books. (Reproduced by permission of the Berkshire Record Office)

By 1900, there were also trades such as carter, cowman, dining hall attendant, shepherd and cook, and the list grew for decades thereafter.

Annual inspections[13] were carried out by the Commissioners in Lunacy (later Commissioners for the Board of Control). Care was taken not to send the same commissioners in consecutive years, although the names repeat over time. The first known female commissioner was Isabel G.H. Wilson, who visited jointly with a

Mr H.C. Devas on 10 July 1935. Their reports were handwritten in heavy, bound volumes labelled 'Visitors Book', which were also used for the signed statements by members of the Committee of Visitors, declaring that they had carried out their monthly duties of touring the hospital and satisfying themselves that all was in order. These books inform us on the major affairs of the establishment, although the author craves the reader's indulgence if any of the sometimes erratic script has resulted in misspelt names or misunderstandings. The tradition of mysterious handwriting seems to belong to those involved in healthcare.

Falling Below Par

The Commissioners' inspection reports show that the asylum carried out its work diligently and, for the most part, effectively but there were usually troubles below the surface. Although always expressed in the most gentlemanly terms, there were clear concerns that the hospital was – at times persistently – rather backward in its facilities, fittings and equipment, creature comforts and even attitudes. Certainly, Superintendent Murdoch was not fond of change, stating in 1900 that he considered it disturbing for staff and patients alike.

Notwithstanding the repairs, redecoration and replacements that were usually in hand, reports after about 1920 show regular, tactful reminders that the Berkshire Mental Hospital was lagging in such diverse matters as open-air verandahs for TB patients, dedicated admissions wards, sanitary arrangements, writing materials for patients, the provision of a cinema projector and, more importantly, modern diagnostic, treatment and research facilities including X-rays and a pathology laboratory. As late as 1930, the post-mortem room was slated for its unsanitary condition, wooden floor, high autopsy table, lack of hot water and poorly equipped viewing room. By 1938, there was still no admissions hospital 'to bring the hospital into line with modern requirements', the infirmary wards being used instead. Further details will be found below and in the relevant chapters.

Although we must allow that these were hard times, it is difficult to avoid wondering whether Dr Walter Woolfe Read, superintendent of the day, was inclined to be reactionary or whether his Committee of Visitors was excessively careful of expenditure. In mitigation, a Commissioners' comment of 1938, generally recommending 'a stitch in time', made it quite clear that costs were indeed an inhibitory factor.

The Commissioners deserve credit for recognising effort and improvement where this was warranted but one report clearly states that the hospital was well below the expected efficiency standard in 1921. This was reiterated in a 1926 report that applauded 'new lighting, new heating, new fire appliances, new water supply, new laundry machinery, new disinfecting arrangements, new bake house fittings, external and internal redecoration and improvements in clerical accommodation – a brief list but one containing works of great magnitude and utility …' but the list

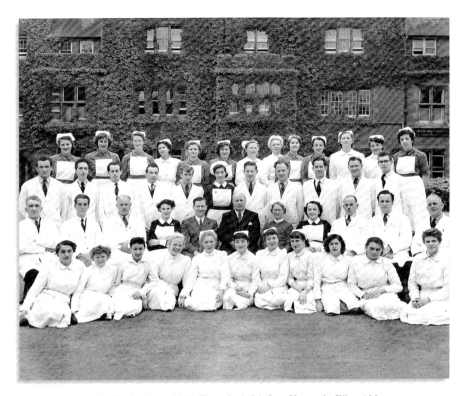

A staff group under Dr Ogden, *c.*1958. Rear, far left is Lou Kennedy. Ellen Abbott
(German maiden name unknown) is 3rd from right. Standing, third row, from left: 6th May
Lehaney (later Walsh); 7th Bill Keating; 9th Joe Hughes. Seated: 1st Martin Brennan; 2nd Lem
White; 3rd Bill Brough; 5th Harry Lambert, Chief Male Nurse; 6th Superintendent William
Ogden; 7th Matron Agnes Pilgrim; 8th Edie Meatyard; 9th Rumney; 10th Idwyll John.
It is believed that Matron Pilgrim retired at about this time. (Bill Nicholls)

of required improvements never seemed to shorten and the kitchen (detailed in
Chapter 3) was a target for heavy criticism for many years.

The National Health Service Act of 1946 – surely one of the world's most
enlightened pieces of legislation – brought changes in the hospital's control and its
final change of name, to Fair Mile. Berkshire Mental Hospitals Group Management
Committee was created in 1948 as part of the NHS and sat within the Oxford
Regional Health Board until 1974. The committee became known as the St Birinus
Group Hospital Management Committee, probably in 1968 when local mental
hospitals were regrouped. It managed two hospitals for the mentally ill, of which
Fair Mile was the larger, and five institutions for those with learning disabilities.
The Commissioners' visits, which have contributed so many insights to this history,
continued until at least 1968, the date of the most recent entry held at the Berkshire
Records Office (BRO).

The final phase in Fair Mile's administrative history is summed up succinctly by
the following quotation from the National Archives:

Under NHS reorganisation in 1974 mental health and learning disability services across Berkshire were managed by the Oxford Regional Health Authority, and from 1994 they were managed under various local NHS trusts including the West Berkshire Priority Care Services NHS Trust, East Berkshire Community Health Trust, and East Berkshire Learning Disabilities Trust. In 2001 these were brought together in one body responsible for mental health and learning disability services called the Berkshire Healthcare NHS Trust.

INFRASTRUCTURE

....

Howell's designs for the Moulsford Asylum were based on careful consideration and much experience; it followed the pattern of his previous asylums in being broadly self-sufficient and providing a good level of comfort and wellbeing for its occupants. This required some of the most advanced technology then available, covering heating, sanitary arrangements, catering facilities, water supply and lighting. It cannot be said that all these innovations were immediate successes and much had to be repaired or modified over the ensuing decades. Behind the purely structural arrangements followed a long list of on-site facilities that kept the hospital operating by producing clothing, bedding, bread and cakes, footwear and a host of other necessities, as well as tending to horses, farm animals, repairs and installations, stores of equipment, raw materials and provisions.

Most of the major functions of the asylum are described under the following headings.

Boilers

As the heart of the establishment, the boiler room had an involved history that we can only glimpse here.

Coal-fired boilers for hot water and steam-pumping engines were an early feature. The original boilers are believed to have been supplied by the Reading Ironwork Company, since this firm was charged with making repairs or improvements over the years, parts being 'returned' to Reading in some instances.

As the asylum was enlarged to meet demand, it was necessary in 1898 to plan for a new and much larger boiler house adjoining the original, to the north of the main frontage. In service in 1900, this was a substantial affair, accompanied by a tall brick chimney and flanked by its attendant coal yard, battery room, engine house, workshop and – supervision of the boilers being a twenty-four-hours-a-day affair – a bedroom for the stoker. Electric lighting was installed at this time, an innovation that caused much ado in the boiler house and warrants its own account later in this chapter. Electricity also powered machinery in the laundry and kitchen.

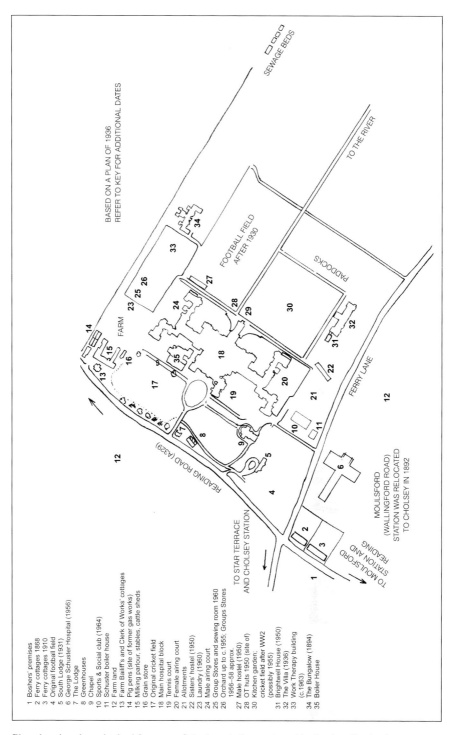

1　Boshers' premises
2　Ferry cottages 1868
3　Ferry cottages 1910
4　Original football field
5　South Lodge (1931)
6　George Schuster Hospital (1956)
7　The Lodge
8　Greenhouses
9　Chapel
10　Sports & Social club (1964)
11　Schuster boiler house
12　Farm land
13　Farm Bailiff's and Clerk of Works' cottages
14　Pig pens (site of former gas works)
15　Milking parlour, stables, cattle sheds
16　Grain store
17　Original cricket field
18　Main hospital block
19　Tennis court
20　Female airing court
21　Allotments
22　Sisters' hostel (1950)
23　Laundry (1960)
24　Male airing court
25　Group Stores and sewing room 1960
26　Orchard up to c. 1955; Groups Stores
　　1956–58 approx.
27　Male hostel (1950)
28　OT huts 1950 (site of)
30　Kitchen garden;
　　cricket field after WW2
　　(possibly 1955)
31　Brightwell House (1950)
32　The Villa (1936)
33　Work Therapy building
　　(c. 1963)
34　The Bungalow (1894)
35　Boiler House

Plan showing the principal features of the hospital over time. (Author's collection)

Pipes and cables for water, gas and electricity reached the asylum buildings through a network of underground service passageways. These were said to flood at times and most were filled in when Fair Mile became a housing development.

The boiler house was situated at the front of the asylum for logistical reasons, including delivery of coal and the proximity of the wells. It stood alongside the cricket field, where it was screened from the pleasure grounds by trees and shrubs. Over the years, the boiler house chimney was raised to lift its smoke to a suitable height, although it was also later reduced in stages.

Records for June 1887 show that the purchase of a Steam Roarer (a loud steam whistle) at a price of 50*s* was requested through the Committee of Visitors, for the purposes of raising a general alarm. This was part of a request for a range of fire-fighting measures and came hot on the heels of a chimney fire in one of the wards. After the Second World War, the Steam Roarer was replaced by a whistle with a far less agreeable sound, which many Cholsey residents remember shattering the calm at frequent intervals – not always at socially acceptable hours – to announce the escape of a patient or as a prelude to the distant two-tone horns of the Wallingford Fire Brigade, which was summoned to false alarms with almost tiresome regularity.

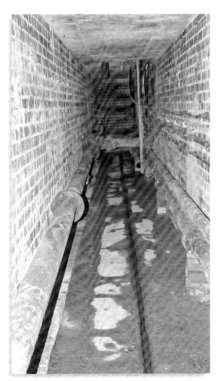

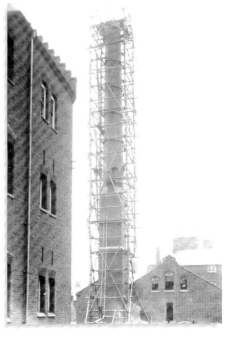

One of Fair Mile's many service tunnels. (Bill Nicholls)

The large new boiler house and its chimney under construction in 1900. Male 6 is on the left. Note the insulators for the newly installed telephone line. (Rod Wilkins)

STOKER BRIGNALL

Ernest John Brignall was born in 1872 and in 1895 moved from Bromley in Kent in pursuit of the position of Stoker at the Moulsford Asylum. He brought good references but was small of stature, which gave rise to

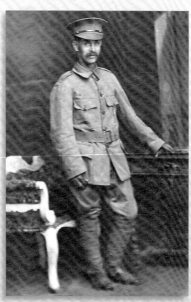

comment at his interview. In reply, Ernest replied that he could get anywhere that the big men could, and many places that they couldn't. He got the job and remained in it until his retirement in 1932.

At the asylum he met Alice Wells, a doctor's maid, and married her in 1897 before setting up home in Cholsey. He was a provident and thoughtful man and, despite his humble occupation, succeeded in buying his own cottage with extensive gardens and orchards, where he could indulge in his hobby of bee-keeping, surrounded by his large family. Mr Moses Nicholls, steward of the asylum from 1881 to 1922, took a benevolent interest in the little stoker, lending him money to help buy the cottage and seeing to it that the repayments were within his means.

Stoker Ernest John Brignall in Volunteer Training Corps uniform in about 1915. (Vera Wheeler)

The boiler house provided 'pressure treatment' for sterilisation. This would have been a high-pressure steam process, commonly known as autoclaving, which had been invented in 1879, although the earliest discovered reference to this being done on site is from 1935.

In 1960, three new oil-fired boilers were installed and considerably automated. The 1956 George Schuster Hospital boasted a compact boiler house of its own that worked away discreetly on the southern side of the main site.

Coal and Coke

Solid fuels such as coal for the boilers and gasworks were essential commodities that were regularly mentioned in the minutes of the Committee of Visitors. As for all major purchases, competitive quotations were requested. Among a number of similar accounts, an entry of 16 April 1909 records the acceptance of tenders

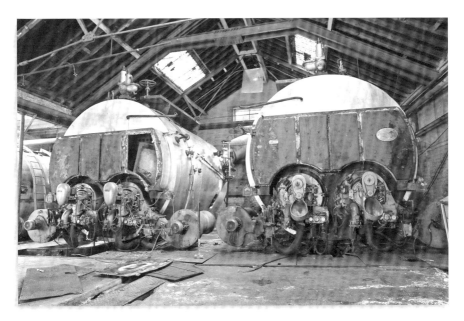

The 1960 boilers in 2010. (Bill Nicholls)

for Wallingford Gas Coke at 17*s* 6*d* per ton from Snow & Sons, Wallingford; also Powell Duffryn (Aberman) Large Steam Coal at 20*s* 5*d* per ton. In addition to this, the Great Western Coal Co., Reading, was to supply 'up to three trucks of samples of Cannock & Rugeley Cobbles at 16/6 per ton; Eveson Coal & Coke Co., Birmingham, to supply up to three waggons of samples of Chapel End Spires Cobbles at 18/5 per ton'. The colourful naming of varieties of coal is intriguing and we should probably assume that 'samples' amounting to several wagonloads were actually paid for.

Water Pumping

Rainwater harvesting, now a fashionably 'green' technology, was designed into the hospital's buildings from the start and the soft water pumped up to large cisterns for use in the laundry. Drinking water initially came from two wells within the main building but two Weir steam pumps later drew it from boreholes up to 100 feet deep, to guard against drought and to ensure that fires could be fought. Those who, in their youth, glimpsed the steam engines that drove the pumps and generators recall that they were visions in gleaming red paint and polished steel, sitting in a pit and immaculately maintained by the Engineer and his assistants. The boreholes were beneath the old cricket pitch, and this supply was in use long after mains water arrived in about 1935. The standard of the water came under scrutiny at times in connection with enteric diseases. Although one shallow well was condemned, analyses regularly found the water commendably pure; first-hand accounts say it was delicious and sweet-tasting. With evident displeasure, Mary Fairbairn, mentioned in Chapter 10, recalled being made to drink the new chlorinated water as part of her training in 1936.

Piped water was originally distributed from a dignified water tower in the front range and later from a tall, steel water tower alongside the boiler house. The steam pumps gave way to electricity as part of a wave of modernisation following the Second World War. Local folklore has it that the electric replacements failed to raise the water as efficiently as steam had done.

Gas Lighting

Given its large and lofty interior spaces, the asylum could not have operated effectively without the significant Victorian[14] development of gas lighting. But mains gas was not available until 1952 and a dedicated gas works was part of the 1870 scheme, located by the north-eastern boundary on the farm site. All seems to have been well enough in its early days but one superintendent's reports mention a number of incidents showing that gas-making was not entirely trouble-free. In April 1886, for example, Robert Bryce Gilland reported the total loss of the gas supply, plunging the asylum into darkness and no doubt making proper supervision of the patients very difficult. The problem was traced to the improperly fitted cover of a purifier, which had allowed all the gas to escape. Gilland's report is notable for his enlightened concern over the risk of explosion and the safety of the Engineer and the Gasman, who was a skilled employee.

Coal gas (specifically 'illuminating gas') is produced by heating coal and capturing the flammable vapours that are given off. The gas then has to be purified to remove contaminants such as coal tar, ammonia and hydrogen sulphide. Gilland's last report, in October 1886, contains the isolated and somewhat cryptic comment 'The gas supplied is very bad at present', suggesting either that insufficient was available or that it contained noxious impurities.

Having given up his position at short notice because of failing health, Dr Gilland's baton and burdens were taken up by Dr John Barron, Acting Medical Superintendent, who reported in December that there had been trouble with the 'gas bar' (an obscure term but clearly a piece of purification equipment), which was overflowing into the boundary ditch and killing the hedge. Replacement was put in hand but, properly watchful of the asylum's finances, Barron tried in vain to find a purchaser for the old one and was reduced to suggesting that it might have to be given away to anyone prepared to remove it, as it was '… becoming a nuisance in its present state'.

The young Dr Joel Harrington Douty had taken up his appointment as Superintendent in time to preside over major renovations to the gas works in April 1887, which included a second gas holder. An enlarged purifier shed was finished in July after delays caused by poor-quality materials. Good news was recorded in May, when the installation of more efficient burners permitted a 20 per cent reduction in the gas pressure and consequent cost savings. It was mentioned that the Recreation Hall, which had previously been gloomy, was now well lighted.

Into each life a little rain must fall for, the following August, Douty was obliged to dismiss Hill, the Gasman, for drunken insubordination. An advertisement for his replacement was duly placed, quite possibly in the *Journal of Gas Lighting*, at a wage of 18*s* per week plus accommodation, rising to £1 after a year.

Electric lighting made the gas works redundant in 1900 and local maps show that it had been removed by 1914.

Electricity

There being no mains supply, the asylum had its own steam-driven generators, which initially supplied power for machinery only, since lighting was still by gas.

Bringing the newfangled electric lighting to such a large establishment was both farsighted and fraught with technical challenges but, proposed in 1898 and switched on with due ceremony on 3 October 1900, this innovation figured in George Thomas Hine's major improvements (see Chapter 4). There were three steam-powered dynamos but their output was not always adequate. 'Extra windings in the field' would hopefully remedy this. The exhaust steam from these, incidentally, heated the hot water supply.

There was also a battery of 110 lead-acid accumulators that supported the system at night, when generation was at a low level. By 1910 the system was under review and the accumulator system had been declared unsatisfactory. The committee solicited expert advice on installing 'new electric engines' from Mr Walter Binns of the Reading Tramways Co. Mr Binns' counsel resulted in the authorisation to purchase, from Messrs Browett Lindley & Co., Manchester, a steam engine and 110 volt DC dynamo at a cost of £216 7*s* 6*d*, inclusive of a maker's written guarantee for twelve months.

This move triggered a series of deliberations that would prove costly. In November 1911, two existing steam engines[15] were found to be inadequate for the proposed task and a new one had to be considered. A subcommittee was duly set up to ponder the issue.

By March 1912 there had been further consideration of lighting plans, discovering that the boilers might now need upgrading before satisfactory performance could be expected from the engines and dynamo, and it was noted that over £2,800 had already been spent on aspects of the boiler equipment in the last year. June 1912 saw Binns recommending a new steam-driven generator of 30kW capacity and sale of the old plant. In the light of technical advances, he also advocated more efficient lamps that would significantly reduce the amount of power that the generator was required to deliver.

Mr Binns presented two reports on boiler efficiency and recommended improved, self-stoking furnaces to guarantee double the steaming efficiency. The carefully selected lamps should reduce the required electric lighting power by two-thirds; the reserve battery was to be replaced with a smaller one and the old would be sold for its lead (although in a later, vicious-circle development, a larger battery had to be considered to support an electric fan that assisted the new furnace).

That October, just as these issues were being overcome, it was found that the boilers were bulging under the increased steam pressure and needed strengthening. The final insult was the discovery of damage to the boilers caused by limescale and impurities in the water. Water softening plant was recommended at the bargain price of 1*d*–1¹/₂*d* per 1,000 gallons after the cost of equipment. This was ordered from Paterson Engineering Co. Ltd, London, for £107 for installation. The boiler repairs went to Hodge & Sons of Millwall for £325.

Shortly after this, Mr Walter Binns went abroad to work and, for his pains, remuneration of 75 guineas was authorised by a grateful Committee of Visitors. It would surely be unjust to suppose that poor Binns was trying to escape the long-winded tribulations of the asylum boilers. At any rate, his improvements lasted until 1923, when we learn that various electrical installations were renewed. Further rewiring was undertaken around 1949, a process that dragged on into 1952, hindering widespread refurbishments that had been prompted by much tactful complaint from the Commissioners.

The modern world is certainly fortunate to have ubiquitous mains electricity; meanwhile the Berkshire Mental Hospital continued to generate its own power until 1954.

THROWING A LITTLE LIGHT ON THE SUBJECT

It is worth bearing in mind that efficient and reliable light bulbs took time to develop. Early types used filaments made of carbonised paper, slivers of bamboo or fine strands of pure carbon. It seems to be the latter that Mr Binns replaced with 'metallic filament lamps of good make' and these were early forms of the tungsten types that are now regarded as inefficient. Hospital records of August 1912 show that these were bought from the General Electric Co. under the familiar name of Osram[16]. They produced 16 candle-power and drew 1.25W per candlepower, making a total of 20W. Given that they were less efficient than present-day 20W bulbs[17], their price of 2*s* 3¹/₂*d* each was high for the modest gleam they must have cast. Even so, among other advantages, we should take it for granted that they outperformed gas lighting by a handsome margin.

Plumbing and Sewerage

In keeping with building codes of the 1850s, the asylum was built with flushing water closets, which were no doubt intended to benefit the health of its occupants. Effluent was pumped eastwards for settlement in sewage beds some way beyond the 1894 Isolation Hospital. After filtration, any liquid run-off was discharged near the river, the flat marshland along the bank being instrumental in preventing any untreated sewage entering the Thames.

In 1872, Superintendent Gilland had to report that the toilets were less than ideal. By 1884, lead pipes had furred up and drains discharging into open grilles were creating a stink, leading to much renewal of pipework, replacement of the WCs and the installation of stench pipes. Twenty-two years into the asylum's life, in May 1892, Superintendent Douty reported continuing trouble with the drains, complaining of sewer gas ingress and lack of ventilation in some of the toilets. In October, he proposed doing away with the troublesome cesspools, even though mains sewerage did not reach Cholsey until the 1950s. In an effort to narrow down the cause of enteric illnesses, bans were placed on the use of sewage as fertilizer and, for trial periods, the growing of vegetables was itself banned. Regrettably, the toilet arrangements repeatedly came under scrutiny as possible causes of diarrhoea, enteric fever and typhoid.

The problem of outdated plumbing was among the longest-lasting found in the records and, in July 1954, Visitors Donnison and Morrell were moved to describe some of the sanitary blocks as 'prehistoric'.

Centralised Heating

Although hot water from the boiler house was available for washing and heating from the asylum's inception in 1870, the science of central heating was as yet immature. The archives suggest that heating equipment was initially distributed around the ward blocks and the chapel certainly had its own stove. There were 'dry furnaces' in the wards, supplying warm air through ducts but these may actually have been the 'auxiliary heating' mentioned in journals. The eminent firm of Messrs Haden of Trowbridge was the main heating contractor and there is strong evidence that it was a piped hot-water system – but perhaps not fed from a single boiler. Owing to continuing marginal performance, Hadens were enjoined to make numerous improvements and replacements at minimum cost.

An entry of October 1872 may illustrate at least part of the problem, it being a request from Superintendent Gilland to be allowed to have the hot-water tanks and pipes lagged, using 'hair-felt and Leroy's Non-Conducting Composition' to remedy a shortage of hot water on bathing days. At times, the heating was incapable of warming the patients' accommodations above 60° Fahrenheit (below 16°C) during bitter winter weather. Less to be expected was Superintendent Douty's 1887 complaint that the post-mortem room was intolerably cold.

Although fireplaces had been built into the wards, they were more for appearance than function and, from 1887, the situation was exacerbated by coal rationing through the use of coal boxes. In August 1892, an agreement was reached with Haden's on improvements to the heating system, which were still not entirely effective. A report the following January recommended laying a complete new main to the Female Hospital Ward at a cost of £49 plus £40 labour.

The complete centralisation of the heating was a conspicuous and welcome feature of Hine's alterations of about 1900, when the larger boiler house entered service although, by May 1910, Haden's were recommending relaying parts of the heating circuit and other changes. They also recommended a very futuristic-sounding 'Turbo-Accelerater' (*sic*) at £62; the work was to be completed by September.

Heating difficulties recurred sporadically, with the Ministry of Health becoming involved in inspections in 1924, and even in November 1933 the Commissioners were expressing the hope that radiators would not completely supplant fires, for reasons both aesthetic and practical: the hospital was still not over-warm.

The subject of hot water for washing and bathing is of course closely allied to central heating. Despite hot water being piped into the washrooms during the 1900 improvements, connection to the basins was apparently an optional extra. Worse still is the knowledge that 'full hot & cold' was not universally available until the hospital had existed for over sixty years. Commissioners' reports throughout the 1930s lamented this deficiency, along with the antiquated and often unsanitary state of the washbasins. As mentioned above, the deficient and dilapidated state of the 'sanitary annexes' and washrooms appears to have been an insuperable problem.

Laundry

The laundry was a substantial installation on the Female side of the hospital and women were encouraged to assist with the work. In the absence of automatic machinery, the workload of washing clothing and bedding for upwards of 300 patients and staff must have been very heavy by 1875. The laundry acquired a ferocious-sounding 'steam calender', or powered mangle, in 1897 but, despite increasing amounts of equipment being electrically driven via a shaft beneath the floor, washing was still done in wooden tubs. Spilt water ran away through the flagstone floor into the underfloor space, which led to evil smells and unsanitary conditions, so by 1901 the floor was ripped out and replaced with one that was solid and waterproof. At the same time, earthenware tubs replaced the wooden ones. With up to 800 patients to serve, Hine's improvements covered rearrangement of the laundry and the installation of steam-heated, fan-assisted drying closets, a washing machine, boiling coppers and a 'hydro-extractor' (spin dryer), all powered by a single 20 horsepower electric motor.

The laundry remained the most mechanised part of the hospital, even if the apparatus was basic, and the safety of workers was a legitimate consideration. The Visitors pointed out in 1912 that the wooden covers of the wringer were unsafe and 'iron net work covers hung with counter balancing weights' were recommended. The same equipment, this time referred to as 'the calender' came under scrutiny in 1934 for lack of protection against accidental injury. This exactly reflects the supposedly modern health and safety doctrine of 'machinery guarding'.

Such improvements do not mean that all was now lavender-scented and blue-white, for it must be remembered that any hospital laundry faces particular challenges relating to the spread of infection. (See page 42.)

New hydro-extractors arrived in 1937 and, in the same year, the Commissioners tactfully suggested that 'a steam trouser press either in the laundry or the tailor's shop would be of value in improving the appearance of the male patients' clothing', but by 1938 they were insisting that, despite these and a new foul washer, a new laundry would have to be constructed to meet demand.

This timing was unfortunate, for war was brewing and we can assume that the public purse was all but padlocked in the face of national uncertainty. Fast-forward to 1956, when the weekly workload was now some 28,000 articles, and the situation was seen as desperate. In an all-too-familiar pattern, the facility was forced to soldier on until 1960, when it was relocated to a new building at the south-east end of the farm complex and connecting with the stores and the sewing room beyond. The old laundry was demolished, to be rebuilt as a desperately needed, new and enlarged hospital kitchen.

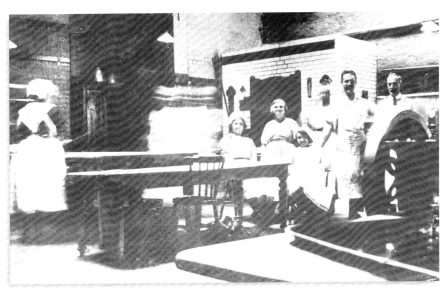

The laundry in about 1900. Note the electric lighting. The blurring is due to staff moving about during a slow exposure. (Spackman collection)

THE POWER OF STEAM

In March 1931, the Commissioners made an observation that may have had far-reaching consequences – that 'foul linen' (meaning bedding soiled with faeces and/or urine) was disinfected only by passing through the washing machine – and tests were duly ordered. Further, it was noted that the wheeled bins used to transport the dirty linen from the wards were sanitised only by dipping them in disinfectant. Commissioners Hopson and Williams suggested using a steam jet instead and this advice was followed, although there is no clear indication that the equipment had arrived until at least the spring of 1932. Subsequent reports suggest that outbreaks of enteric fever, typhoid, dysentery and the like became much less frequent; no further mention is made until 1941, when an outbreak of paratyphoid fever was confined to a single ward.

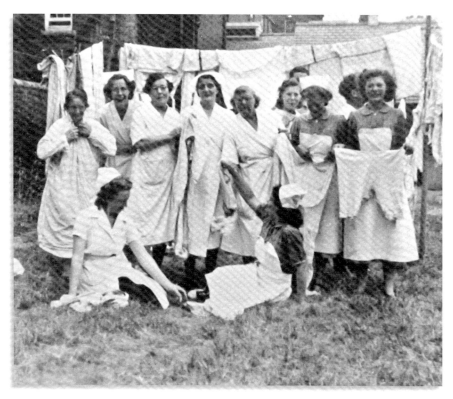

A lighter moment among the laundry and domestic ladies, late 1940s. Standing, from left: Ada Blissett; Jessie Matthews; Mrs Wallis; Mrs Heath; Marion Matheson; Rosie Marshall; Doris Marshall; others unknown except far right ? Groves. Seated: Lena Birnie and Lynna Ganz. (Spackman collection)

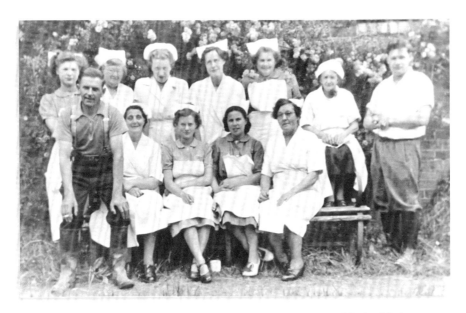

Laundry and domestic staff, late 1940s. Standing, from left: ? Groves; Marion Matheson; Lena Birnie; possibly ? Jones; Joan Woodward; Ada Blissett; Sid 'Paddy' Patrick. Seated: Chris Ruttle; Mrs Heath; Rosie Marshall; Lynna Ganz; Mrs. Wallis. Chris Ruttle was the lifelong companion of Joan Woodward, who was in charge of the laundry and very popular. Chris and Sid Patrick worked in the laundry despite their Wellington boots. Marion Matheson was known to many as 'Aunt Marion'. (Spackman collection)

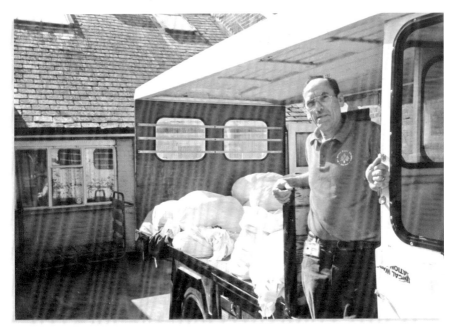

Michael 'Wacker' Strange delivering laundry bags to the wards in 1992. (Spackman collection)

Kitchen

Very little descriptive information about the hospital kitchen survives, most references being concerned with staff changes, dietary patterns (see Chapter 6) or complaints about structural problems. It was originally situated near the back of the central block, behind the administrative offices and stores, adjacent to the dining hall.

Meals were at first cooked on coal-fired ranges or else steamed, gas cookers not arriving until 1880. The gas works produced insufficient volume for cooking, and was done away with before 1914, so electricity from the asylum's powerhouse is likely to have taken over as the energy source. Mains gas was piped to the kitchen when it became available in 1952.

There were hints of trouble to come in a 1926 report. After complimenting the hospital on a long list of improvements, the Commissioners were moved to comment, very tactfully:

> ... we hesitate to do more than draw attention to the inadequate character of the kitchen accommodation ... We would suggest for consideration the possibility of the adoption of the system of ward feeding throughout the hospital and the consequent liberation of the present dining room for conversion into kitchen accommodation.

There is no indication of any improvement by about 1930, although an electric mixer appeared at the behest of the Commissioners. Refrigeration was slow in arriving for a hospital of any kind: in 1936, the Commissioners commented on its absence and that the meat room was full of flies. Since there was apparently no money for a refrigerator, the cheaper installation of gauze doors and windows was suggested. In May 1937, the safety-conscious Commissioners had to report, 'We noted in the kitchen the need for adequate protection of the bacon and bread cutting machine. Its condition yesterday was dangerous.'

By December 1938, it was apparent that an extension and re-equipping of the kitchen were essential. There was insufficient cooking capacity for the hospital's growing population and, for want of steamers, puddings could be provided only three times a week. This was written in tones of urgency, yet the following year's report made the astute observation that improvements to both the kitchen and laundry might have to be delayed in the face of wartime restrictions.

Superintendent Hugh Astley Cooper and the Visitors were keenly aware that the roofs of both the kitchen and laundry had become positively dangerous by October 1940. They also received criticism of the storage of perishable foods in ward kitchens, especially when sick cases were in the ward. Refrigerators were now essential and there was brief mention that these could be had in either electric- or gas-powered form, even though there was no gas supply. A more basic and achievable target was the provision of breadboxes.

Another year on, we see that, as a fuel-saving measure, 'In contemplation [is] the installation of a large slow-combustion cooker & two boiling pans in the main kitchen.' This hints at solid fuel and was actually delivered within the next twelve months. Meanwhile, repairs to the roofs of the kitchen and laundry were still wanting, and were causing real anxiety.

War or no war, on 24 July 1943 the Commissioners went to town, declaring the kitchen to be in a disgraceful state:

> We know that a number of the Hospital Committee realise that the kitchen is obsolete. In fact this department is one of [the] most unsatisfactory we have seen in a mental hospital. Since the erection of a new kitchen or thorough reorganisation of the department is impracticable during the war period, discussion for the present has to be restricted to minor improvements. The Committee we understand have under consideration improving the ventilation of the central portion of the kitchen where the boilers and steamers are situated. When this is done we hope that the cleaning and redecoration of the walls will be undertaken, so as to ensure better hygienic conditions.
>
> The kitchen is stuffed liberally with both paid workers and patients; we feel that with more supervision of these workers and a little more system, conditions in this department would be improved materially even in the present circumstances.

It is not clear what this tirade actually achieved; the October 1944 inspection suggested only that bread in transit to the wards should be covered with cloths as lidded metal bins could not be provided, presumably because metals were largely prioritised to munitions and aircraft.

Following earlier reports of unexplained shortfalls, all patients were at least now on full civilian rations and a specimen meal of cold pork, pickles and baked rice pudding met with approval. Meal planning was almost invariably considered to be good, although somewhat at the mercy of available supplies.

With the end of the war finally in sight, the July 1945 Commissioners' report expressed satisfaction that there were now rooms for storage and cutting of bread, and took particular pleasure in the arrival of tin containers with covers for transporting it. A 'steam canopy' (extractor hood) had also been fitted in the kitchen and work had commenced on stripping the walls, which were subsequently sprayed with asbestos. Progress perhaps moves in mysterious ways.

More equipment arrived during 1947 but rats and mice had by now augmented the kitchen's woes and a replacement was still the only solution, which even the new NHS could not provide; in 1955 the kitchen's condition was dreadful and replacement depended on relocating the laundry (see above). There was the same annual story of apparent inaction until at last, in 1960, the old laundry could be gleefully demolished to provide a suitable site. Almost three more years elapsed before,

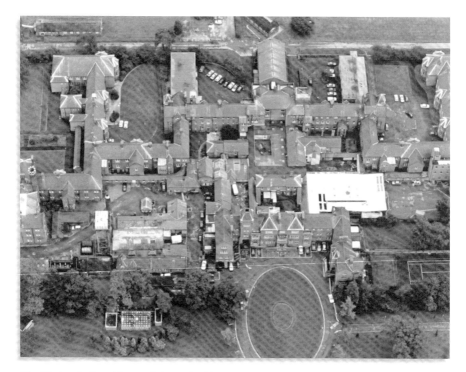

The kitchen is the white-roofed area in this 1990 view from the north-west. Note also the pump houses over the old boreholes, lower left, and the two rectangular wings of 1957, flanking the Recreation Hall. (Spackman collection)

in 1964, we first hear of the extensive, white-roofed and completed facility that produced meals for the remainder of the hospital's life. As if to prove a point, there was immediate trouble with the flooring.

Bakery

The asylum's bakery keeps a very low profile in the archives but we know that it was enlarged by Howell in 1881. With 800 mouths to feed by 1902, it is gratifying to learn that Hine doubled its size and equipped it with a kneading machine powered by a 6 horsepower electric motor! Baker's yeast was an essential commodity, delivered at frequent intervals; in the late 1930s, the van was marked 'DCL'.[18]

Farm and Gardens

By 1871, around fifty patients were regularly helping to produce foodstuffs on the asylum's farm. Reports of about 1900 to the Commissioners in Lunacy show large quantities of milk, cream, butter, eggs, poultry, beef, mutton, veal, pork, suet, potatoes and vegetables being produced and accounted for by value. The farm had a stock yard, calving and farrowing pens, stables, a milking parlour, cart sheds and a slaughterhouse. Heavy horses provided the motive power, requiring stabling and mucking out; the dairy herd was served by a resident bull and the piggery produced pork that was sold to Wall's, the pie and sausage concern. Grain was harvested and threshed for storage on site, while the straw was required for animals' bedding. Mangolds were grown for animal feed in the large field to the south of Ferry Lane, and parties of male patients would go out to do the hoeing and harvesting, sometimes enjoying beer brought to them in large jugs.

Horses continued to provide motive power until after the Second World War and were replaced by tractors only after 1946. The end of that conflict brought the farm a new and well-equipped dairy, although it was not long before it became easier to buy milk in from outside.

Peace saw a slow decline in the farm's importance and areas were taken over for use by transport and other services. The piggery was still active in the late 1970s but the farm closed not long after Mr Edward Smithers, manager since 1946, retired in 1975.

Neither the kitchen garden nor the orchard was in place when the asylum opened. Dr Gilland reported on 20 September 1872 that his sketch plan for a kitchen garden had been approved, and it was staked out during the following month. The square plot, situated behind the Female wards, was divided by a cruciform network of paths, clearly

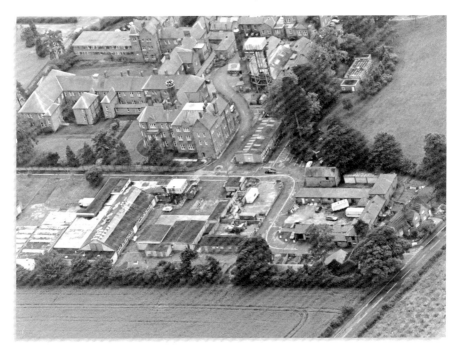

The farm site in about 1990, now much altered. The laundry and stores are bottom left, with transport centre and remnants of the farm to the right. The cottages occupied by the Farm Bailiff and Clerk of Works stand by the road. (Spackman collection)

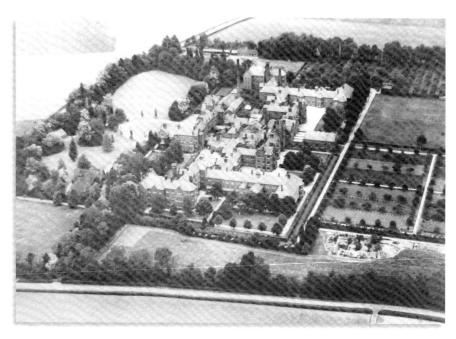

The kitchen garden (centre right) and the orchard (top right) are well portrayed in this *c.*1927 photo, while the greenhouses can be glimpsed centre left. The large grassed area upper left was the original cricket field. Ferry Lane runs left to right towards the Thames. (Spackman collection)

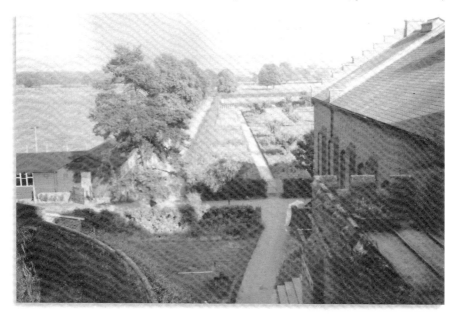

A glimpse of the kitchen garden from Renee Gorman's room near the Recreation Hall, in 1951. The garden was turned into a cricket field soon afterwards. The path leads down to the river. Note the high wall of the airing court, bottom left, and the wooden Occupational Therapy huts. (Renee Brewerton, née Gorman)

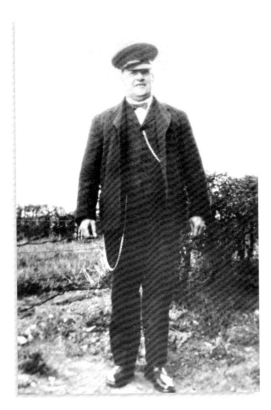

This attendant was identified as Charlie Crean, a former New York policeman who supervised outdoor working parties, although the dating evidence does not support this. The uniform is typical of around 1932. (Spackman collection)

FARM LAND

The asylum originally rented agricultural land from the wealthy Morrison[19] family of nearby Lower Basildon but in 1911 the Morrisons were selling off parcels of land, with existing tenants having first option. The asylum was offered nearly 89 acres at £35 per acre. The Committee of Visitors inspected the land and notified agents Rawlence and Squarey that they were prepared to offer £25 an acre. Rawlence and Squarey sportingly responded that they might consider £30. Rarely keen on parting with money, in November 1911 the Visitors instructed their clerk to reply that £25 was all they would consider. Messrs R. & S. were not impressed.

There was a notable lack of comment on the matter in December's meeting but in January 1912 we find a slightly sheepish note that, following complicated calculations, it had been decided to pay £30 per acre, subject to financing the purchase over fifty years. This went ahead in April 1912, but not before the cost-conscious Visitors had learnt that, under the provisions of the Local Government Act, 1888 *et al.*, they were prevented from borrowing money over a period greater than thirty years.

GIANT CABBAGES

In the BMH period, the establishment still made full use of its sewage beds, the management of which fell to one or more male patients, who apparently made a good job of it. Through fortitude, enterprise and the addition of farm manure, valuable nutrients were recovered for the greater good of the hospital's productive fields and gardens.

In the 1930s, Lilian Talbot, former nurse and by now wife of the Hall Porter, appreciated her allocation of home-grown vegetables as much as any young mother. One day, when a particularly impressive cabbage was delivered to her door, she insisted that it be changed for something smaller, since she was aware that someone was growing them on the walkways between the sewage beds!

visible in the photograph on page 48, and fruit trees were planted among the vegetable beds; this produced a pleasant place for patients to work. An extensive orchard was established between the south-east of the farm and the later isolation hospital.

The kitchen garden's healthy potato crop warranted mention in Dr Gilland's early journals and staple vegetables such as carrots, cabbages, sprouts, parsnips and leeks were still cropping during the Second World War, supplying the hospital kitchen and those members of staff whose wages entitled them to a share, who received deliveries twice a week in a large basket.

Greenhouses

Heated greenhouses stood just to the south of the lodge cottage and produced flowers for the wards, plus a variety of hot-house fruits and vegetables such as tomatoes, cucumbers and melons. Mr Henry Last was Head Gardener from 1906 until 1938 and became skilled at this form of horticulture; yields were good enough that luxury items like asparagus, although grown for the doctors and senior officers, would sometimes reach ordinary members of staff. During the war, the post of Head Gardener was held Mr Bill Chamberlain.

Pharmacy

The hospital had its own pharmacist but the department drew little attention to itself. Its final home was in rooms built in 1881 and 1901 as mess and recreation rooms for male staff. The opening of the social club building in 1964 probably made this space available.

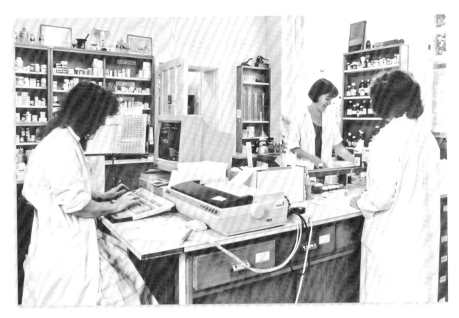

A 1980s view of the pharmacy. Ruth Ellenby on left and Katy Sims centre.
(Spackman collection)

Stores: Old, New and Newer

The General Stores originally occupied a relatively small area in the central block of the asylum building and kept nearly all of the asylum's supplies and spares.

Items that could not be produced on site were put out to tender and the lists make interesting reading. Although extensive lists of bought-in provisions can be seen in the Visitors' ledgers, these do not include staple foods, which probably came under the control of the Steward.

Other items, such as those listed in September 1909, included black lead, boiled mutton, oatmeal, starch, bath bricks, tobacco, treacle, blacking, hearthstones and extract of beef (Bovril). A Mr F. Wheeler of Wallingford supplied soda and salt. In February 1912, among other clothing and fabrics, E. Jackson & Sons of Kings Road Corner, Reading, supplied tapestry carpet, hearth rugs, men's neckerchiefs, men's felt hats and '24 gross black dress buttons'.

It is remarkable that the stores remained in such small quarters until after the Second World War. Peace and progress brought many more proprietary items and new ways of thinking. Thus a much larger, purpose-built stores was erected in 1956 on part of the former orchard, lying alongside the boundary hedge. This boasted large windows and an impressive roof of sheet asbestos; an electric delivery vehicle was procured to deliver goods around the site. Sadly, the building went up in flames a few years later. No precise account seems to exist but anecdotes say that the place 'burned like a Roman candle' and that roofing sheets exploded like bombs in the intense heat.

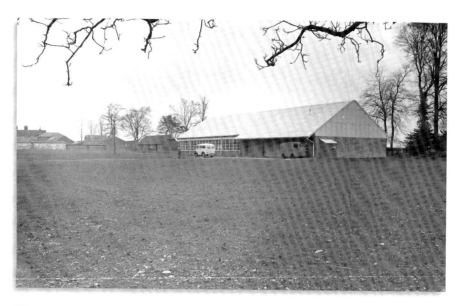

The 1956 Group Stores building. Note the farm site beyond. The site was previously the large orchard. (Spackman collection)

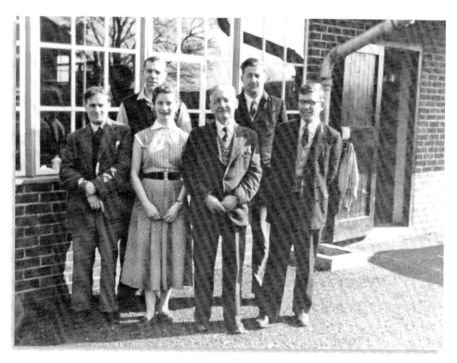

Staff outside the new Group Stores in 1956. From left: Vic Whittick, storeman; Frank Rowswell; possibly Miss Shaw or Beryl Smithers; Gerald Woolley; Laurie Blake; Mick Broad (driver). Woolley was in charge of stores and Blake was his second-in-command. The stores burned down after a very short life. (Spackman collection)

The replacement – and final – stores of 1960 stood at the edge of the farm site, parts of which had by now been taken over for other uses. It incorporated the linen store and connected with the laundry and sewing room, which were put up alongside and operational in May of the same year.

Communications

We are nowadays helpless without telephone or email, undreamt of in 1870. Instead, an electric bell system was installed at least as early as 1872, with which the asylum could summon staff living in nearby Star Terrace. In 1887 this included the Head Male Attendant, Mr Alfred Lockie. A note in the margin of Superintendent Douty's first report in that year reads 'Add means for return ring', suggesting that it would have been useful to know whether anyone in Star Terrace was paying attention.

The telephone arrived in 1900, doubtless a great boon to the senior officers and soon taken for granted, for little further is recorded about telecommunications, apart from re-equipment in 1923. It is an interesting aside that, until about 1970, all Cholsey numbers consisted of just three digits!

Patients' Workshops

A range of gainful activities not only gave patients a purpose but reduced the net cost of running the asylum. Some worked out of doors, some in the laundry or kitchen and some tended the wards, but the April 1904 ground plan on page 14 also shows us that workshops were in place for tailoring, boot-making and cobbling, dressmaking and mattress stuffing. Although the assistance patients could render was often small, this was nevertheless a part of their therapy.

Unfortunately, we know relatively little about the long histories of these shops. Recruiting a resident bootmaker was an early challenge for Superintendent Gilland, but his journal records success in December 1871, when Simion Lyford was hired, to be assisted by five working patients. Robert Townley arrived as Assistant Shoemaker in 1885, while Harry Lammas was Shoemaker from 1911 to 1943. Henry Aldborough was hired as Tailor in March 1872 and there can be little doubt that he was also assisted by patients who would, among other tasks, recover buttons from worn-out clothing.

Hair picking, which was the sorting and untangling of horsehair for stuffing mattresses, is one of the few activities mentioned in the official reports. This dusty task was probably also rather itchy and it is scarcely surprising that, in 1929, it was suggested that a lean-to or shed would be more suitable than an indoor workshop. Mattress stuffing was clearly a major enterprise, producing goods for Fair Mile and other institutions at least until 1949.

The sewing room and tailor's shop between them produced or repaired much of the hospital linen (all with sewn-in ward numbers), uniforms and patients' everyday clothing, and female patients turned out quantities of aprons, night attire, flannel drawers, dresses, shirts, socks and stockings. Until about 1935, clothing tended to be serviceable at the expense of high style, but some items were bought in. The division

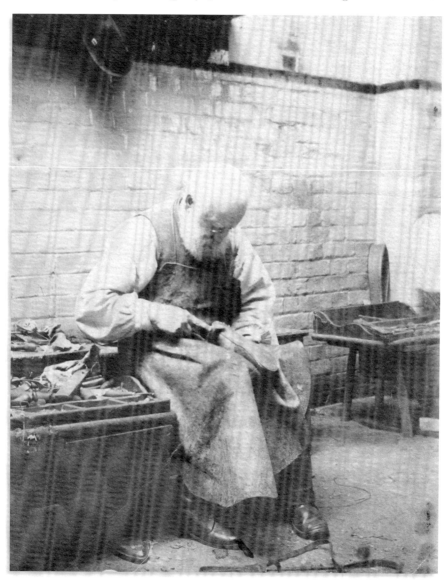

This atmospheric study is thought to be of Mr William Watts, a Wokingham patient who suffered from depression, in about 1910. Another patient, a Mr Warburton, an artist who had been exhibited at the Royal Academy, produced a superb pencil rendering that survives in the author's family. (Spackman collection)

of the sewing room in the late 1930s, to afford facilities for Occupational Therapy, presumably reduced the overall output of clothing. On the other hand, the women gained the opportunity to select and make their own clothing, which must have been beneficial overall.

For many years there was an upholstery workshop alongside the boiler house, which saved huge expenditure on furniture. The Commissioners' report of 1935, when the shop was run by a Mr Ivermee, relates that wicker chairs were being upholstered for the greater comfort of patients. The last known location of the workshop was in a shed close to the farm.

Complete figures are not available but it is recorded that 66 per cent of patients were employed in gainful work in 1899; in 1936 there were forty women in the laundry, another sixty to seventy in the sewing room, and a large number of men working in the farm or the grounds. This is not a sound comparison but appears to be a much smaller proportion of the total of 859 souls then resident.

Pathology and X-ray

At the start of 1926, there was a strong recommendation that a pathology laboratory be set up (or else arrangements made with another hospital) to investigate the causes of death, disease and epidemic. As in so many other areas, progress was so slow that one has to entertain the possibility of reluctance on the part of the hospital's officers. In 1929, Commissioner Herbert C. Bailey wrote:

> I hope the time is not very far distant when this hospital will be equipped with
> an admission hospital and a treatment centre with those modern appliances,
> such as X-rays, violet rays, continuous baths[20] and other things which are now
> so generally used as aids to the successful treatment of mental troubles.

No laboratory was in prospect by 1932 but the end of 1938 saw official satisfaction at the conversion of a disused ward kitchen – yet this may never have been completed as the shortcoming is repeatedly mentioned up to 1942, when a small laboratory existed in Male 2. Notwithstanding, pathology was being done at the Royal Berkshire Hospital – not at Fair Mile – in 1951.

X-ray facilities fared no better; those for TB at least were still being done at Reading in 1948, and the results reviewed by the County Tuberculosis Officer. Not until 1949 did work start on a radiological unit, which required its own diesel generator. When it opened in 1950, it was operated by technicians based in Reading.

In fairness to all – given the strictures of wartime and the consequent huge increase in the hospital's patient population – the following statement, dated 22 May 1946, by Commissioners W.S. Mackay and H.C. Devas, does much to deflect any blame from Superintendent William Ogden and the Visitors:

There is much to do to raise this hospital to the standard of up to date efficiency which it will undoubtedly achieve. There is no need to mention in detail all the needs. The facts are well known to the Committee and Superintendent and we were much impressed by what is being done and the amount of thought that has been given to detailed planning for the future. It is regrettable that in present circumstances progress is bound to be slow. Many of the plans are inter-dependent and must follow a sequence, for example the provision of a nurses' home, which is the most urgent necessity at the moment, will release accom-modation for badly needed clinical rooms and other purposes; the building of an admission hospital will enable the wards at present used for this purpose to be used for the more satisfactory care of patients with tuberculosis for whom the present arrangements, particularly on the female side, are poor: a new staff dining room will allow provision of a proper lecture room for nurses and a sit-ting room for male staff; it will also allow the operating theatre to be used solely for its original purpose. It is unfortunate that there are no satisfactory quarters for married medical officers.

On the positive side good progress is being made with redecoration of wards and reconstruction of sanitary annexes. The farm has been brought up to date and is a pleasure to see. A new herd of tuberculosis-tested cattle has been started. More important is the development of the clinical side, particu-larly the out-patient and child guidance work.

After two years in a country that was at peace with most of the rest of the world, Commissioners J. Coffin Duncan and R.G. Anderson recorded in late 1947 that slow inroads had been made into improvements and there was praise for what had been achieved. It was understood that 'present difficulties' (almost certainly the nation's impoverished post-war state) prevented rapid progress. A significant defi-ciency was in staff housing.

Dr Ogden had done what he could to improve staff amenities, for example a new mixed staff dining room by the kitchens and a new male nurses' sitting room; female nurses now had two sitting rooms in the 1870 superintendent's residence, although they needed refurnishing, rugs and lighting. There was also a lecture room for the new Preliminary Training School. Nevertheless, wards were still being described as drab, needing redecoration and comfortable furniture; easy chairs were most urgently needed. Some staircases were dangerously worn and liable to cause accidents.

As the National Health Service era approached, a report penned in July 1948 by Commissioners Coffin Duncan and Anderson lamented the slow pace of urgent improvements, but was again charitable enough to record that Ogden was fighting an uphill battle and that his difficulties were understood by the Board of Control. There was still no admissions hospital; no convalescent villas; overcrowding and the time-worn problem of staff shortages. Adding difficulty was the presence of about

150 people with learning difficulties who, it was appreciated, should be cared for at a specialist unit. These poor souls, added to a wartime influx from Hill End and Brookwood Hospitals, represented an overload on the nursing staff the hospital had managed to recruit or retain.

The Mortuary

This was situated on the west wall of the boiler house from at least 1904. The building was part of the original boiler house complex and it is not clear whether the mortuary was always there. A young Vera Talbot and her little brother, John, who lived in the Lodge, one day couldn't resist climbing up to look in through the window – and rather wished they hadn't. There are few mentions of the mortuary in the archives and, hardly surprisingly, no detail of the solemn proceedings it hosted.

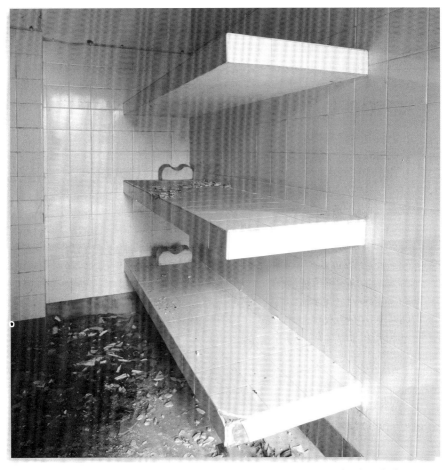

The mortuary was a small building adjacent to the boiler house. It housed a chapel of rest, a refrigerator for three corpses, a post-mortem table and these shelves. (Bill Nicholls)

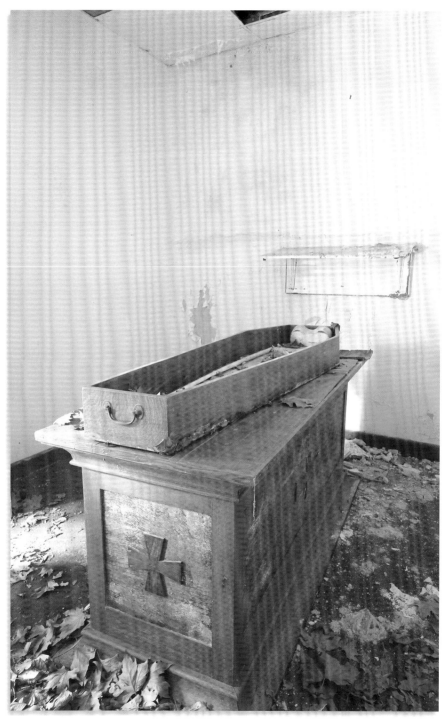

The tiny chapel of rest adjacent to the mortuary. These forlorn views are from 2011.
(Bill Nicholls)

4

EXPANSION

....

More or less chronologically, here is an account of the significant enlargements to the asylum over many years.

Four staff cottages standing along the Reading Road perimeter were all in place for the 1870 opening of the Moulsford Asylum. Tenure of each was associated with a particular responsibility; for example, in the early 1930s, the semi-detached cottage at the gate to the asylum's farm was occupied by Mr William (Bill) Southby, Clerk of Works, and his wife. The adjoining property was that of Mr Chris Carter, Farm Bailiff from 1897 to 1946. A hundred yards to the south, by the main gate, stood the lodge cottage, which was assigned to the Hall Porter, Mr Leslie Talbot and his family, whose neighbours were Mr Last, Head Gardener, and his wife.

Unsurprisingly, the arrangements for staff accommodation were supplemented and altered over the asylum's long history, according to the needs and fashions of the day.

Star Terrace

Although some believe that Star Terrace, in nearby Papist Way, was built for the asylum's use, it was in fact purchased from the estate of a Mr Bowler in 1872. The cottages, on three floors, were described as 'newly built' and the auctioneers were quick to point out

Have received Instructions from the Trustees of the late Mr. W. Bowler,

TO SELL BY AUCTION,
AT THE STAR INN, CHOLSEY,
(ADJOINING THE PROPERTY)

On Friday, January 19th, 1872, at 3 o'Clock in the Afternoon,

In Five Lots. Subject to Conditions of Sale to be then produced and read.

LOT 1

A FREEHOLD BRICK BUILT & TILED COTTAGE,

Containing Front Sitting Room, Kitchen, 3 Bed Rooms, Washhouse, Outbuildings & good Garden.

LOT 2 TWO SIMILAR COTTAGES
„   3 TWO DITTO
„   4 TWO DITTO
„   5 TWO DITTO

These Cottages are newly built, and are the nearest Buildings to the new County Asylum at Moulsford.

For further Particulars apply to Messrs. Morland & Son, Solicitors, Abingdon, or to the Auctioneers, East St. Helen's, Abingdon.

M. EVANS, PRINTER, ABINGDON.

(Reproduced by permission of the Berkshire Record Office)

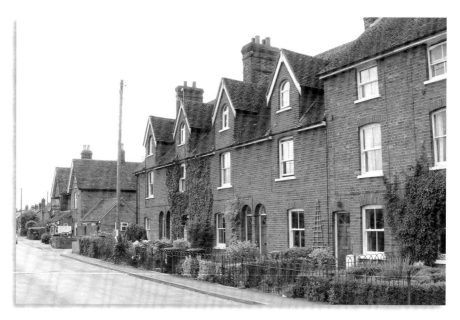

Part of Star Terrace and the neighbouring Morning Star pub. (Author's collection)

that they were 'the nearest buildings to the new County Asylum at Moulsford'. Money changed hands on 25 September 1872, a deposit of £90 representing 10 per cent of the purchase price. Although Star Terrace usually housed artisan staff such as the farm hands or upholsterer, Alfred Lockie, Head Male Attendant from at least 1875, had one cottage, while Mr Porter and Mr Matheson, both attendants, and Perce Talbot, stoker, were there many years later. The terrace is now in private hands.

Howell's Extensions, *c*.1881

Almost as soon as it had opened, Dr Gilland found himself faced with heavy demands on the asylum's capacity. The majority of its 285 beds had been filled within twelve months of opening and were all occupied by May 1875. Meanwhile, Berkshire continued to use its allocation at Littlemore but in 1876 Oxfordshire, with troubles of its own, took steps to buy out Berkshire's places. This precipitated urgent expansion at Moulsford, again supervised by C.H. Howell and, between 1878 and 1881, 400 additional beds were made available by adding Male and Female wards 4 to 7. The hospital plan on page 14 is based on a 1904 drawing by Thomas Dinwiddy & Sons, which claims an original 200 beds, plus the 400 new. Whatever the exact figures, demand exceeded supply and *Change at Cholsey – Again!* tells of 'patients sleeping on the floor until new beds were bought to go in the corridors'. The new building work included additions to staff accommodation outside the site, extension of the chapel, a recreation hall and improvements to infrastructure, notably the laundry and bakery.

The Recreation Hall

This was part of Howell's 1881 scheme and adjoined an extension of the dining hall at the rear of the asylum. Although plain and described by some as rather small, it had a large stage with rooms beneath and an excellent dance floor. Naturally it was the social centre and the scene of many dances, concerts, pantomimes and parties. When its huge sliding doors were rolled back the combined dining room and hall made an impressive space.

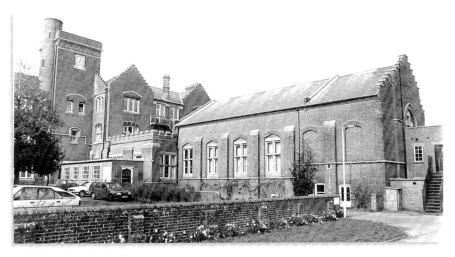

The 1881 Recreation Hall in about 2000. The castellated roofline beyond marks the contemporary extension of the dining hall. Note the projection room at the extreme right. (Spackman collection)

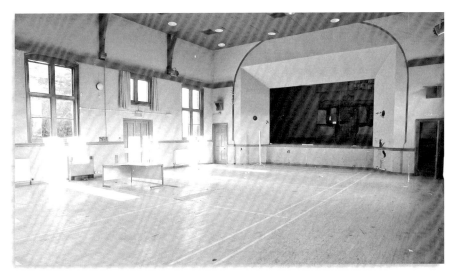

The Recreation Hall or 'Great Hall' before restoration. Note the false ceiling. The panelling around the stage had protected many original features. (Bill Nicholls)

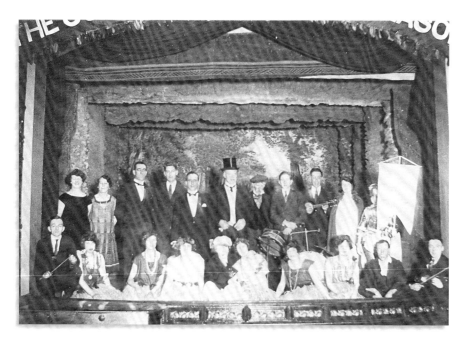

The banner over the stage of the Berkshire Mental Hospital's Recreation Hall appears to read 'THE COMPLIMENTS OF THE SEASON', suggesting a Christmas show. The date is estimated at 1930. Ray Beasley is 8th from left, then Roddy Hutt and Vi Hearmon. The violinist on the far right may be Alf Alsopp, charge nurse, who also played trombone with Cholsey Silver Band. (Spackman collection)

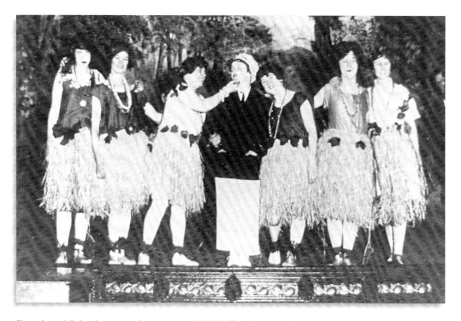

Dancing girls in the same show around 1930. (Spackman collection)

The Isolation Hospital

To combat the spread of dangerous diseases, an isolation hospital was built in 1894, costing £2,879. The single-storey building stood by the north-eastern perimeter, well removed from the main blocks. The architect was George Thomas Hine, RIBA, like Howell a specialist in asylum architecture. Tuberculosis affected the asylum

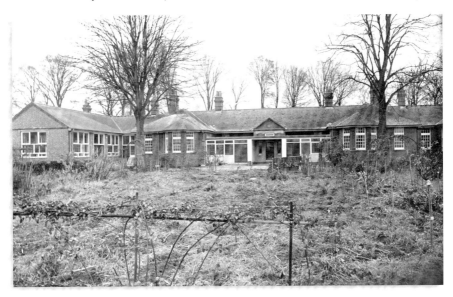

The Bungalow in the 1960s. The gardens are not at their best. (Spackman collection)

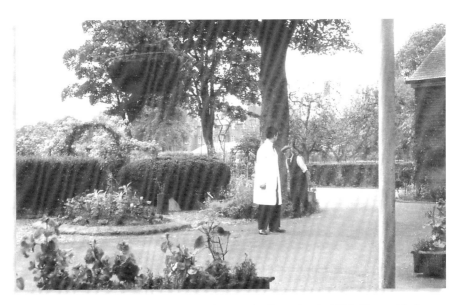

Renato Zito and an unknown patient/gardener at the Bungalow in 1958. (Renato Zito)

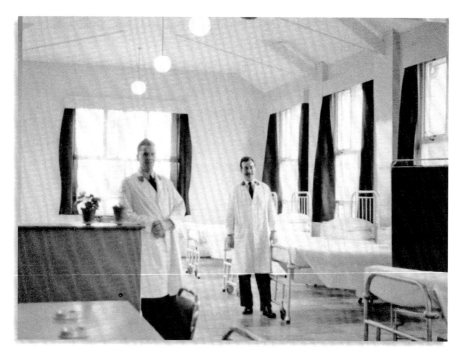

Dick Nicholls and colleague in the Bungalow, *c*.1950. (Bill Nicholls)

for many years and was among the principal reasons for this addition, which staff and even official reports called 'the Bungalow'. Surrounded by attractive gardens and screened by trees, it was a peaceful retreat. Extensions and alterations made in 1929 accommodated fourteen extra patients. With improvements in the treatment of previously intractable diseases, consideration was given in 1935 to assigning it to low-supervision male patients on the same basis as in the Villa (see page 69), although the Commissioners noted that it was still 'admirably used for debilitated or tuberculous female patients'. From the 1970s, the unit was officially Rotherfield Ward and at various times it was used as a secure unit and by the hospital's forensic service. Sadly, the Bungalow did not survive the hospital's redevelopment.

Hine's Extensions, *c*.1900

Having been obliged to relinquish its own arrangements with Littlemore, the Borough of New Windsor joined the Bodies in Union in 1896, adding to pressure on ward accommodation at Moulsford. In 1898, George Hine submitted plans for two new two-storey wings with 100 beds apiece – housing Male and Female wards 8 and 9 – a further extension of the chapel and bakery and the new boiler house that provided centralized heating and generated electricity. Electric lighting replaced gas and a telephone system was installed, while some existing wards received interior panelling.

A contract for groundwork and foundations was awarded to Benfield and Loxley of Oxford, and completed by April 1899, while the upper works went to Parnell & Son of Rugby. Sadly, there were delays associated with one of the service tunnels and a shortage of facing bricks. This had the superintendent expressing his frustration in March 1900, since the weather was ideal for building. A year later, only sixteen new beds were available and overcrowding was unavoidable until the new wards could be opened in 1902.

Ferry Cottages

Two rows of staff houses, usually called Ferry Cottages, stand along the Reading Road to the south-west of Ferry Lane. One of these is believed to have been built at the same time as the asylum and to have housed building workers before allocation to nursing staff. The house nearest to the asylum was usually allocated to the Head Male Attendant; around 1900, this was Mr Jack Woolley and, from 1936 to 1952, Mr Jack Croxford, who was in turn replaced by Mr Harold Lambert.

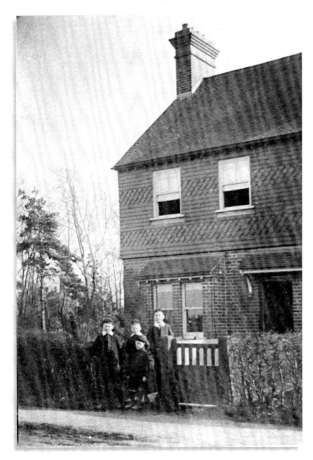

Jack Woolley was Head Male Attendant when this view of No. 1 Ferry Cottages was taken in about 1906. His son Gerald (far right) later managed the stores and married Annie Kirk, pictured in Chapter 10. (Spackman collection)

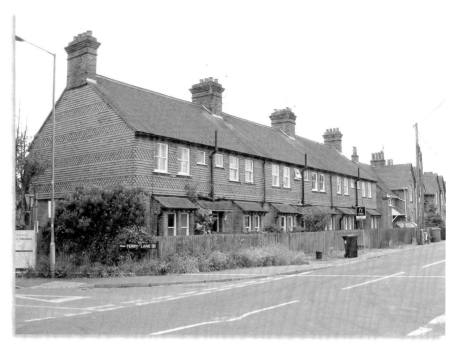

The *c.*1870 terrace at Ferry Cottages, pictured in 2014. (Author's collection)

A second row was proposed in 1911, the architect being a Mr W. Roland Howell – no obvious relative of C.H. Howell. The design incorporated cost-saving features, such as a split-level layout that followed the contours of the ground. When asked, in rather lofty tones, why the designs incorporated earth closets, the practical Howell pointed out that there was little alternative, since no sewer was available. His considered view was that earth closets were healthier than cesspools and that the gardens were large enough that the soil could be dug into them.

The extremely local firm of Boshers – directly across the Reading Road – submitted the lowest tender to build all six cottages for £1,657 8*s* 9*d* but the Committee was sold on the idea of spending only the £1,460 estimated by Howell and ordered reductions in the specification to achieve this, such as cheaper bricks and plaster, deleting a soakaway, thinner doors and gravel paths instead of paved. As this did not produce the desired result, Howell was paid for his services and a different architect engaged.

The cottages were finally approved in April 1911 at a cost of £1,662 17*s* 3*d*, but suffered protracted problems from leaking roofs, which may prove that you get what you pay for.

Boshers' unrivalled proximity may have won them numerous other contracts, such as South Lodge, Brightwell House, alterations to various wards, the Work Therapy building, new kitchen, extension of the sports and social club premises and a new roof for the George Schuster Hospital, most of which are mentioned below.

South Lodge

The medical superintendent originally enjoyed a four-storeyed residence attached to the south-west frontage, commanding a splendid view from the main gate to the asylum's front door and having private gardens to its rear.[21] For the superintendent's convenience, the house was connected to the asylum buildings by a curving corridor with a castellated roofline[22], although the corresponding disadvantages of this arrangement can readily be imagined. More to the point, a connecting door direct from the house to the Female dormitories was installed in 1886. The reason for this is unclear but Dr Gilland's final monthly report contains his complaint of much disturbance by noises from the dorm, 'which permeate the entire house'. The castellated outside corridor was demolished some time after 1958: traces of its presence can still be discerned.

Proposed in 1929 and recorded as nearing completion in March 1931, a spacious, modern, detached house was built on land in the western corner of the site, previously used as a football ground. Known as the South Lodge, this was the 'Super's house' for several decades and the original residence was adapted to house twenty-six female patients in an 'open' ward. This had been achieved by 1932. South Lodge later became surplus to requirements and by 1988 was used as a crèche. Meanwhile, the original residence had become office accommodation.

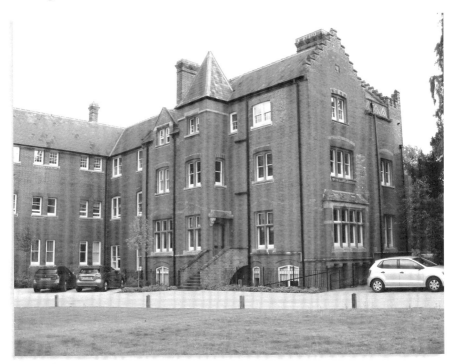

The 1870 superintendent's residence, restored and once again a home in 2014. Note repairs to the end wall, following removal of the fire escapes. (Author's collection)

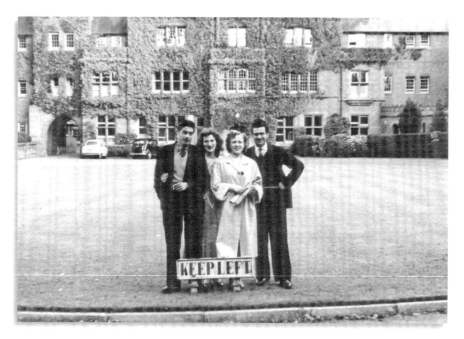

Italian student nurses De-Bin Artemio, Antonia Cassella, (unknown) and Renato Zito on the Oval in 1958. Note the original shape of the arch to the left and the castellated corridor on the right. (Renato Zito)

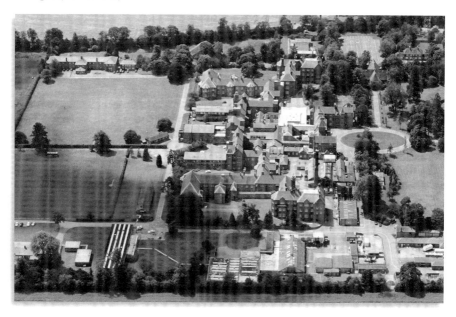

Ranged left to right along the near boundary are the Bungalow, Work Therapy, Stores (roughly centre), Laundry and Transport, with the remains of the farm at the right. The Villa and Brightwell House are top left and South Lodge upper right. (Spackman collection)

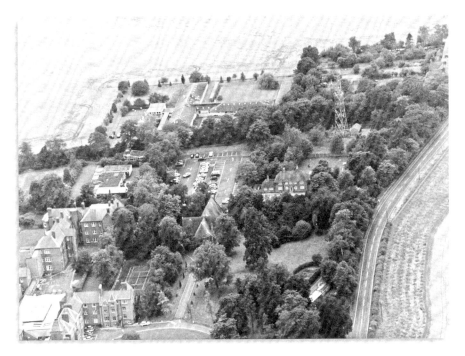

South Lodge is centre right. The Schuster is in the distance and its boiler house can be seen just above the sports and social club premises, which are to the left of the car park. We also get a glimpse of the heated greenhouses near the A329 Reading Road. (Spackman collection)

The Villa and Brightwell House

In 1933, the decision was made to construct a detached ward block alongside Ferry Lane. It was to accommodate 100 female patients who did not require the close supervision of the main hospital, and who consequently enjoyed considerable freedom. From the outset, this large building was known as the Villa.[23] Progress with construction was slow, as observed in November 1934 by the Commissioners, who expected it to open in January 1935. By July of that year, it was said to be almost ready for furnishing and expected to open in September, yet it was not until the first week of July 1936 that forty-eight female patients 'of well-behaved chronic type' had moved in. In 1941 it had to be divided into two wards, later known as Kintbury and Lambourn, to help cope with a wartime influx from another hospital. Brightwell House, built at the same time and connected by a passageway, housed the matron[24] and, later, administrative staff.

By the 1970s, declining patient numbers made the Villa available for use as the Newlands Day Hospital. Reflecting new thinking in the form of group therapy, Fair Mile's Winterbourne Therapeutic Community, which opened in 1967 under Chief Psychiatrist Dr David Duncan, moved from the admissions wards (the Schuster) to the Villa in 1975. Day patients – typically suffering from anxiety, stress, neurosis, loss

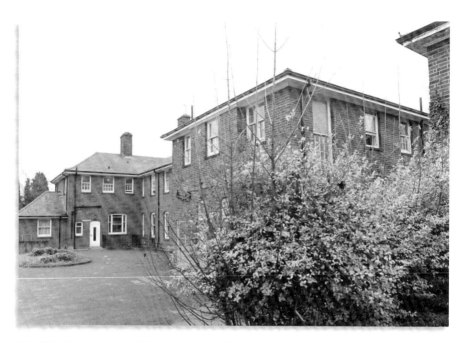

The Villa (Lambourn and Kintbury wards and later the Newlands Day Hospital) in about 2001. (Spackman collection)

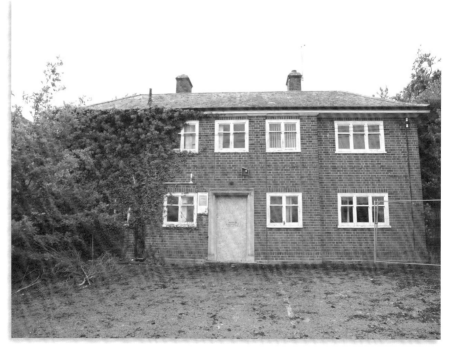

Brightwell House shortly before demolition in 2010. It stood just to the north of the Villa. (Bill Nicholls)

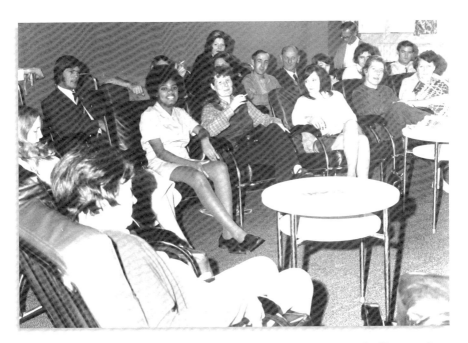

A relaxed session at the Winterbourne Unit in 1972. It was also known as the Therapeutic Community. Charge Nurse Bob Wright is smartly dressed on the left. (Spackman collection)

of confidence, eating disorders or drug problems, rather than a mental disorder – benefited from this approach. The Winterbourne Unit later moved to Moreton ward before relocating to Reading in August 1995 as Fair Mile eased towards closure.

Projection Room

After many years of prevarication, a cinema projector arrived in 1939 and was housed in an ugly, brick room tacked on to the Recreation Hall. The result would nevertheless have been greatly appreciated by patients and staff alike, who could now have access to newsreels and features that were otherwise either out of bounds in nearby Wallingford or inconveniently timed for shift workers.

The Male and Sisters' Hostels

The pressures of the Second World War swelled the hospital's patient population to its peak of around 1,400 plus staff. After the conflict, it was still customary for nursing staff to 'live in' and, anticipating the recruitment drive that followed the war, two utilitarian, single-storey hostels were put up behind the hospital in 1950. These housed fourteen male nurses – mostly trainees and junior ranks – and fourteen Sisters (later including staff nurses). The Male hostel stood behind Male 8, just beyond an access road. During its time, under its official name of Barbrook House,

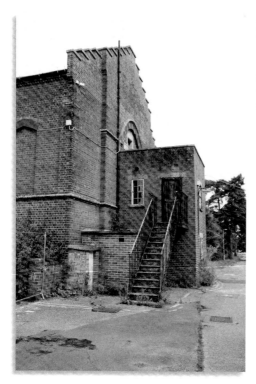

Left: The projection room, no lovelier in 2010 than it was in 1939. (Bill Nicholls)

Opposite: A view of Fair Mile from around 1970, which can be compared with the site plan on page 32. (Spackman collection)

it was unsurprisingly the scene of much mischief but, on a relatively serious note, former male nurse Mike Reynolds tells of a row of poplar trees that stood nearby. One day, a male student was in the hostel toilet, bothering nobody, when one of the poplars crashed through the roof a matter of feet away. The trees were cut down shortly afterwards but the hostel was repaired and served for many more years.

The Sisters' hostel, officially Winterbrook House, was situated rather more privately, a short distance south-east of the main complex and just inside the Ferry Lane boundary. Before long, it had – one must assume fairly – earnt itself the soubriquet The Virgins' Retreat and there was a strict rule that male staff were not permitted in the building after 10 p.m. History has little to say about the success of this policy.

Being cheaply made, the hostels were cold in winter; post-war student nurses can still tell tales of their shortcomings. Although put to other uses, both buildings survived up to the hospital's closure.

The OT Huts

To vacate space in the main hospital, Occupational Therapy operated from two wooden huts, arranged in an L shape, near the back of the Recreation Hall. These were put up in 1950 and served until OT moved in with Work Therapy in about 1964.

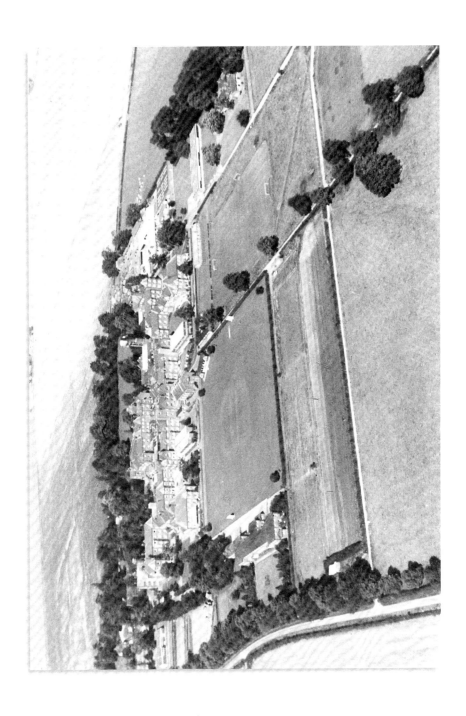

Staff Houses in Papist Way

Other post-war arrivals, in the early 1950s, were two pairs of semi-detached houses, more or less opposite Star Terrace in Papist Way. One of these was occupied by Mr Harper, Clerk of Works, and the others by senior medical staff. One pair was modified in 2000, becoming Cholsey House, a home for nine male patients, which offered a measure of independent living combined with twenty-four-hour nursing assistance.

Bucklands, Whitecross and Chalmore House

The 1947 Commissioners' report observed, for the umpteenth time, that shortage of decent staff accommodation was adversely affecting recruiting. 'No medical officer has a house. The quarters which are available are quite unsuitable for single men of professional standing and far less so for those with wives and young families.' There was still no nurses' home, although plans existed, awaiting an opportunity. In 1952 the Visitors opined that no staff should have to sleep in the side wards.

The hostels (page 71) relieved the pressure to some extent but several substantial local properties were eventually taken over for this purpose. Bucklands, on the Reading Road a mile towards Wallingford, was the first, housing twenty-two female nurses in 1952. Slightly further away and just inside the hamlet of Winterbrook stands Whitecross, then 'A charming country house, capable of development' which, from 1953, was used by eighteen nurses and two assistant matrons. Just outside the centre of Wallingford is Chalmore House, acquired in 1958 for male nurses. These fine properties suffered from being adapted into nurses' homes and Whitecross in particular required extensive restoration when it passed back into private ownership.

The George Schuster Hospital

Many alternatives were used (at one time a sign clearly read George Schuster Ward) but 'Hospital' was the official designation of the long-awaited twenty-four-bed admissions and treatment unit that opened in 1956. For most staff and locals, 'the Schuster' was adequate. New ground was broken on the far side of Ferry Lane, although the Schuster's boiler house stood just inside the Fair Mile boundary. Sir George Ernest Schuster, KCSI, KCMG, CBE, MC was an eminent barrister, financier, administrator and politician who, in 1951, became Chairman of the Oxford Regional Hospital Board. He was concerned that his own wife's depression should be treated in a modern facility and financed this radically innovative building.

The new hospital's architecture, by the distinguished firm of Powell and Moyra, was ultra-modern and raised a few eyebrows in conventional, post-austerity Cholsey. With extensive glazing and a topsy-turvy roofline, it challenged old ideas about the design of healthcare facilities and won an RIBA award.

Part of the Schuster's mission was the treatment of schizophrenics and depressives and it was equipped for the then-fashionable technique of electro-convulsive treatment (ECT). Despite gaining a poor reputation and declining with the advent of better drugs, ECT was valuable and, with refinements, remains an option of last resort.

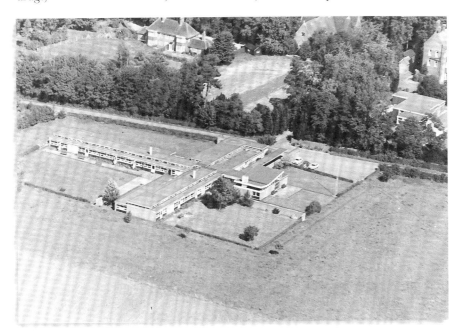

The George Schuster Hospital in about 1970. The Common Room shows off its upside-down roofline. The Super's house is upper left and the Sports and Social Club stands to the right, just beyond Ferry Lane. (Spackman collection)

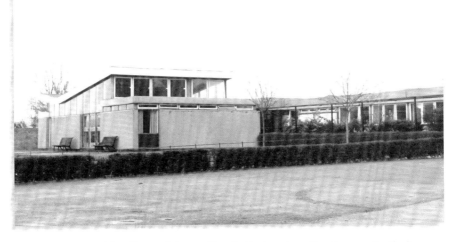

Part of the eye-catching George Schuster Hospital in its prime. (Spackman collection)

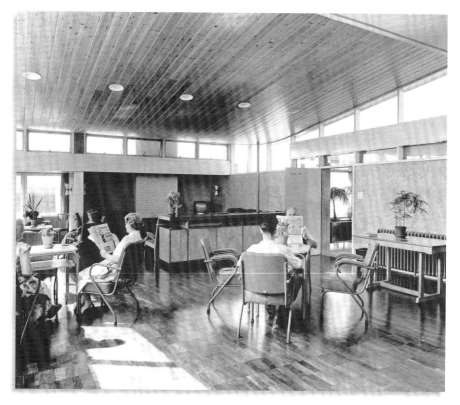

The Schuster's Common Room. (Spackman collection)

The Schuster's interior layout employed long, straight corridors with many doors opening on to them. An informed source pointed out that this kind of scenario is apt to trigger schizophrenic episodes, so it is perhaps fortunate that the building's award was limited to its appearance. The structure did not prove durable, the flat roof leaking through the years 1959 to 1962 and inferior materials causing other problems that culminated in a new roof in 1989. The familiar story of neglected redecoration had left it very shabby by 1967.

Remembered as a happy environment, the Schuster was the first part of the Fair Mile complex to be demolished for redevelopment but did not go down without a fight. Like many 1950s buildings, it was packed full of asbestos, the removal of which halted work for some time.

New Dormitories, *c*.1958

Now well established as Fair Mile, the hospital suffered continued pressure on patient and staff accommodation and construction of two two-storey dormitories was started late in 1957. Their ground floors extended Male 2 (Blewbury) and

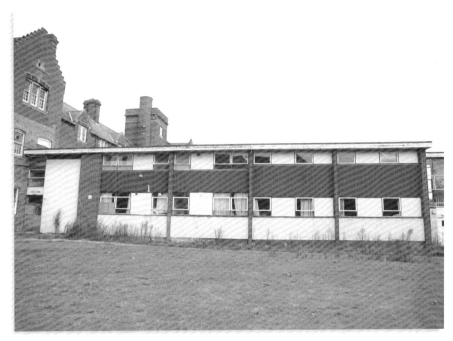

The 1957 extensions to Basildon (ground floor) and Caversham (first floor) wards, admittedly not at their best in 2010. (Bill Nicholls)

Female 2 (Basildon), while the first floors added space to Male 3 (Compton) and Female 3 (Caversham). In common with much of the forward-looking architecture of the time, middle age found them short on visual appeal and they were demolished without ceremony during the redevelopment process, a fact appreciated by the residents of the properties that now overlook their former locations.

Stores, Sewing Room and Laundry

An area lying between the farm and the Bungalow, originally laid to orchards, was grubbed out in 1955 and made the site of a new Group Stores in 1956. It lasted only a few years before burning down. By 1960, its replacement stood nearby, and was connected to the sewing room and the new laundry that arrived the same year. A photograph can be found on page 52.

Work Therapy

After operating in inadequate conditions, Work Therapy and Occupational Therapy jointly acquired a new building in about 1963, on the former orchard site. The north-light roof structure and lack of opening windows caused complaints about overheating.

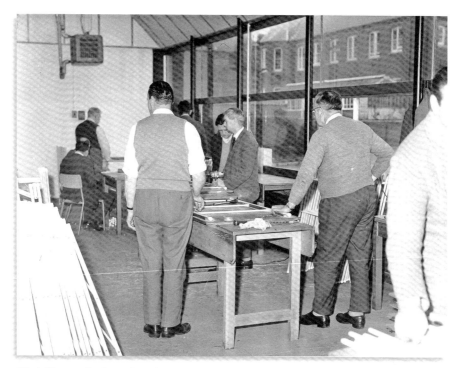

Work Therapy in the early 1960s. The 'sun room' attached to Male 8 (Hermitage) ward can be seen through the window. (Spackman collection)

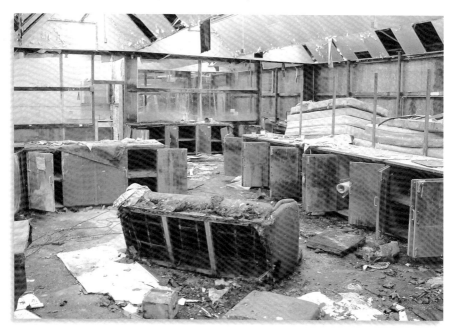

Mattresses stored in the derelict Work Therapy building around 2010. (Bill Nicholls)

5

THE PATIENTS

....

Readers are bound to want to know about the patients, who were the *raison d'être* of Fair Mile, but the fact is that most of the case notes are closed to public scrutiny under the hundred-year rules of confidentiality and those stories that can be viewed would take up considerable space. Also, it is in questionable taste to put anyone's limitations on public display. A limited selection of early case notes can be seen on the Berkshire Record Office's web site www.berkshirerecordoffice.org.uk.

Without being intrusive, let us try to picture the people whose lives were shored up and repaired by Fair Mile's work. If nothing else, this chapter attempts to illustrate the hospital's concern for individuality and dignity.

Although the term 'pauper lunatics' – meaning those without the means to pay for care elsewhere – is little used in the asylum's records, its core objective was their cure. But this was not a free-for-all service; Victorian awareness of the costs involved meant that admission was not granted unless strict criteria were met. Private, fee-paying patients were not admitted until 1872, and then in limited numbers.

The very first page of Dr Gilland's admissions register in September 1870 lists four cases of congenital idiocy; thirteen of dementia due to brain fever, sunstroke, paralysis, epilepsy, intemperance or unknown cause, one of melancholia and two of mania. This is representative of the 111 patients accepted that year and the pattern in 1909 was similar. For many years, patients were classified according to the difficulty of caring for them, rather than their particular illness.

The supposed causes of insanity make interesting reading and an 1882 document lists, among many more predictable sorrows, 'intemperance', 'hyperlactation', 'religious excitement', 'masturbation' and 'the climate of India'. Sad to tell, the curing of the first and last of these did not show a good rate of success.

'Criminal lunatics' were not usually accepted, being normally confined in Broadmoor Criminal Lunatic Asylum at Crowthorne, which opened in 1863 and bore many similarities to the Moulsford Asylum. One early exception to this, in May 1887, occurred when the Secretary for the Home Department arranged for five Pentonville inmates to be received. Much later, a 'secure unit' was set up at the

Bungalow to house an overflow of Broadmoor patients. Local folklore suggests both that they were approaching parole and that the security was not tight enough.

TABLE X.

Showing the probable Causes, Apparent or Assigned, of the Disorder, in the Admissions, Discharges, and Deaths of the year.

CAUSES.	The Admissions			The Discharges. Recovered.			Recovered, Relieved, or otherwise.			The Deaths.		
	Males.	Females.	Total.	Males.	Females.	Total.	Males.	Females.	Total.	Males.	Females.	Total.
MORAL :—												
Disappointment in Love	1	..	1	..	..	..	..	..	..	..	..	..
Family Affairs	..	1	1	..	..	..	..	..	..	..	..	..
Fright	..	1	1	..	..	..	..	..	..	..	..	..
Ill Treatment by Husband	..	1	1	..	..	..	..	..	..	..	..	..
Love Affair	1	..	1	..	..	..	..	..	..	..	..	..
Over Study	1	..	1	..	..	..	..	..	..	..	..	..
Troubles at Chapel	..	1	1	..	1	1	..	..	..	..	..	..
PHYSICAL :—												
Abscess	..	1	1	..	..	..	..	..	..	..	..	..
Accident	1	..	1	..	..	..	..	..	..	1	..	1
Brain Fever	..	..	..	..	..	..	..	..	..	1	..	1
Congenital Defect	10	5	15	..	..	..	..	1	1	..	2	2
Epilepsy	9	5	14	..	..	..	..	..	..	..	..	..
Fever	1	..	1	..	..	..	..	..	..	..	..	..
Fall on Head	1	..	1	..	..	..	..	..	..	1	..	1
Hard Work	1	..	1	..	..	..	..	..	..	..	..	..
Hereditary Tendency	5	11	16	..	1	1	..	..	..	1	..	1
Intemperance	3	4	7	..	..	..	..	..	..	..	1	1
Over Lactation	..	1	1	..	..	..	..	..	..	..	..	..
Puerperal State	..	1	1	..	..	..	..	..	..	..	..	..
Smallpox	..	1	1	..	..	..	..	..	..	..	..	..
Sunstroke	..	..	..	..	1	1	..	..	..	..	..	..
Thunderstorm	..	..	..	..	..	..	..	..	..	1	..	1
Unascertained	51	52	103	4	4	8	1	..	1	8	4	12
TOTAL	85	85	170	4	7	11	1	1	2	13	7	20

TABLE X CAUSES OF INSANITY: an intriguing table of causes of insanity from 1885. (Reproduced by permission of the Berkshire Record Office)

Service Class Patients

Military or 'service' class patients were accommodated in 1923, perhaps earlier, although numbers are not known until 1933, when eighty were present. Seventy arrived from Great Yarmouth in 1940, displaced in the face of wartime priorities. These men enjoyed extra comforts and privileges and the overall impression is that the military normally looked after its own.

Children

Minors with severe learning disabilities were accommodated up to 1930, when Berkshire and Oxfordshire County Councils jointly set up the Borocourt Institution, in nearby Peppard, to provide more appropriate care: however, recognised classes such as 'idiots', 'imbeciles' and 'cretins'[25] were not directed to Moulsford as a matter of course. In 1896, Dr Murdoch complained of having to house hopeless 'congenitally defective, epileptics … demented and aged … idiots and imbeciles'. He was not unsympathetic towards them but felt that the asylums were being used as an easy and unsuitable solution that imposed a burden on his undertaking.

The asylum authorities were generally uneasy about taking in children. In February 1875, an 8-year-old boy from Abingdon was listed as being almost ready for trial discharge. Superintendent Gilland wrote, 'It is very important that he should be sent to school'. A December 1908 entry in the Visitors' minutes contains a resolution that it is undesirable that children associate with adult patients of either sex. Children nevertheless found themselves in the BMH at times; in 1931 Commissioners Hodgson and Adamson noted, 'In Male 8 we saw a boy of 8, a trainable imbecile, who has improved considerably since admission but who should be dealt with under the Mental Deficiency Act and removed to an institution where special training can be afforded.' The most recent instance discovered in this research was in October 1944, when three children with learning difficulties were being cared for. Visitor J.L. Etty commented, 'I am strongly of the opinion that boys of 15 or less ought not to be housed with adult patients'. The reason was a lack of accommodation elsewhere and the Commissioners clearly sought to remedy this.

Geriatrics

Problems associated with old age were handled at the asylum from its earliest days and mention has already been made of feeble souls being transferred from the workhouses, where the necessary support and understanding could not be provided. It is tragic that many of these problems were rooted in malnutrition and the harsh workhouse regime. There is a telling comment from 1926, when sixty-eight out of 146 admissions were from Poor Law Infirmaries and others were from home: 'With regard to the former, we thought that a fair proportion of the senile cases might with adequate nursing have been properly dealt with in infirmaries, without removal to a mental hospital.'

Thankfully, we live in times that address dementia more sympathetically and with better resources.

Voluntary Patients

The Mental Treatment Act of 1930 permitted voluntary admission to mental hospitals, although the available archives make little mention of the subject. In 1936 the Commissioners seemed almost disappointed that the number of voluntary and temporary patients was low, questioning whether GPs and relieving officers '… are not making nearly as much use of the Mental Health Act 1930 as they properly might'. If they were touting for custom, they would have been pleased with the 1939 figure of 25 per cent of cases, any celebration being dampened by curtailment 'for want of adequate accommodation – which is regretted'. Voluntary patients remained a feature of the hospital's activities until its final years, although the proportion was not always as high.

Needless Incarceration

The author has often been asked, or told in general terms, about unfortunate individuals who were confined to a lunatic asylum on the slenderest of pretexts – the first of which is invariably pregnancy out of wedlock. There is an immediate difficulty in answering this question because so many of the patient records remain closed; no evidence of such events has been found to date. What seems more likely is that the unfortunate women were suffering from what we now recognise as post-natal depression or one of the infections that can attend childbirth which, perhaps adding to stress and humiliation, temporarily unbalance the mind. Mark Stevens, Senior Archivist at the BRO, offered his opinion that Victorian sensibilities were robust enough to recognise that 'fatherless' babies are a fact of life. If we also consider the conditions that had to be satisfied before the Bodies in Union were prepared to spend public money on care and rehabilitation, the chances are that instances of families having their errant daughters 'put away' were either exaggerated or very few in number.

Depression, sometimes described as 'laziness', caused individuals to remain at the asylum for extended periods and could be seen as unjust cause for confinement. Such cases could lead to patients becoming institutionalised and losing their ability to cope with the world outside.

The present-day availability of effective drugs and other therapies tends to distort our perceptions of what was considered acceptable and possible a century ago. No doubt future research on the Fair Mile archives will have a few surprises for us all.

Daily Routine

Mary Fairbairn (see Chapter 10) left a description of her ward's weekday routine in the 1930s. This began with day staff arriving at 7 a.m. for breakfast. At 7.30 a.m., after checking dressings, wet beds and suicidal patients, they took charge of the ward from the night nurses, who would have got the patients up and dressed. Patients took breakfast in the Day Room and all the cutlery was counted before they could leave. Medications were issued at 8.15 a.m., after which the ward had to be tidied and cleaned, assisted by those patients who were willing and able.

After 10 a.m., there was time for outdoor exercise or indoor handicrafts and a tea break, before working patients were escorted to the workshops or gardens by Occupational Therapy staff. When they had gone, there was equipment to clean and sterilise and, on visiting days, a change of uniform so as to look fresh and smart.

'Dinner' was at about midday, staff taking their meal at 1 p.m., after which outdoor exercise was again encouraged until 3.30 p.m. Supper arrived at 4.30 p.m. and there was time for newspapers, radio and games while nurses attended to the more needy patients, who were sometimes segregated in the side rooms.

Another round of medications, laxatives, painkillers and so forth was followed at 6.30 p.m. by cleaning and tidying, sorting out the next day's clothes and getting everyone ready for bed at 7.30 p.m., with everything ship-shape in time for the night nurse to take charge at 8 p.m. Needless to say, the night attendant did not always enjoy a quiet time!

Creature Comforts

Luxury was never on the hospital's agenda but decent standards were always desired, if sometimes a little slow in arriving. November 1934 brought criticism of uncomfortable chairs and obsolete beds, hopefully to be gradually replaced. Some of these matters took years to be resolved.

A patients' canteen was opened in 1931 or early 1932 and operated on three days a week, selling tea, sweets, tobacco, oranges and other treats. It immediately proved very popular and was well stocked and well run, attracting favourable comments from the Commissioners. In 1935 they suggested that ice cream would be a good line in summer, perhaps sold on the cricket field. The canteen showed remarkable resilience in the face of wartime rationing, rarely suffering from shortages.

Sweets were popular among those with money to spend, which prompted Commissioner Devas to comment in 1945:

We discussed with Dr Ogden the question of the patients' sweet and chocolate ration, and asked him to consider whether something could be done to ensure that no patient was without sweets or chocolate because of lack of money to make a purchase at the canteen. In many hospitals now the ration is issued free as part of the hospital dietary.

In 1957 there was a suggestion of modest pocket money for just such purposes as this.

The hospital's League of Friends came into existence in 1953 and did much good work to improve patients' lives by funding a range of equipment and indulgences, and by running the canteen on six days a week.

Clothing and Personal Effects

Whilst we don't have much detail of hospital clothing, it is clear that it was functional first and stylish second. Realising that self-esteem was important, the Commissioners were keen to see a change to more attractive apparel. In 1924, Commissioner R.H. Trevor criticised the absence of nightshirts for men and the 'skimpy' nightdresses worn by women, adding that he also thought more slippers should be supplied. The next year, Commissioner Rollisham observed patients in the open air and complained that neither they nor staff were supplied with overcoats. 'This should receive early consideration from the Committee.'

Women patients had a choice of modern styles of clothing by 1935 and could choose their own pattern, made to measure. Undergarments had been similarly updated, either by alteration or replacement. Women also got thinner stockings of various colours. Men were wearing light-coloured socks but it was hoped that dark ones, as worn outside, could be made available.

It is rather shocking to learn that, despite promises to the contrary, patients' underwear was 'pooled' as late as 1959. No doubt the marking, sorting and delivery of personal items was a logistical headache in an overstretched laundry but, out of concern for patients' dignity, this shortcoming attracted just criticism. This apparently did not apply to private patients, who wore their own clothing from at least the 1930s.

Hanging space for clothes, already an established issue, was still non-existent in 1935, even in the newly completed Villa, but was to be provided for some wards. The practice of rolling clothing into bundles at night – overcoats in particular were mentioned – was still normal. During her 1936 visit, Flora Calder, one of the Commissioners, saw bedside lockers for personal possessions in most of the wards and was moved to comment, 'the spectacle of female patients walking in the ward gardens with a bulky bag containing all their small belongings is now conspicuous by its absence.' However, this shortcoming affected male wards into the 1950s.

Men's outfits were moving towards sports jackets and flannels in 1939 and looked smart when ironed. Women's clothes were seen to be attractive and soft but destructive patients still had to wear heavy-duty clothing. The next year, the hospital was criticised for not allowing patients to wear their own clothing, as was the practice elsewhere: laundry difficulties were cited and, given the dire state of the laundry (see Chapter 3), the reason was probably valid.

Personal Grooming

The basics of personal appearance were important but largely limited by the abilities of the nursing staff and patients themselves. A hairdressing salon was installed on the Female side only in 1950. Basic services were free but patients had to pay for perms and suchlike. Meanwhile, the men were still shaved only twice a week, although the Commissioners suggested a minimum of three times.

Complaints

One of the Commissioners' duties was to hear any complaints from the patients; there were typically very few, other than the expected objections to being detained. They regularly commented on the atmosphere of care and consideration for the patients' wellbeing and the cordial relationships between patients and staff, although a few exceptions may be detected in some of the anecdotes offered below.

Outings and Visiting Days

Vera Wheeler (née Talbot) was born and grew to adulthood in the Lodge and has contributed a good deal of information to this account. Here are some of her recollections of the patients from the 1930s and '40s:

> On a couple of afternoons a week, there was what was known as 'the walk'. Patients were taken out – probably between 20 and 30, accompanied by uniformed staff – and they walked from the hospital to the village and back again. Whether they visited the shops – if they had the money to do so – I cannot say. Male patients had their walk on different days … and again, they were supervised by uniformed attendants. I always felt a little sad for these people, and of course a lot of them were left in the hospital because their families did not want them home. Some didn't want to leave; they had been there so long that the hospital was their home, and the staff did their best to make it home for them. I remember one male patient whom I had known for years, got dressed up every Saturday and went to Reading by train, probably to watch football, but eventually it was decided that he really should be discharged. He was distraught … took himself down to the river via Ferry Lane, where there were plenty of people about, and laid himself down in the shallow water at the bottom of the lane. Someone raised the alarm; a member of staff collected him and, after a short time back behind locked doors, his life resumed as it had been for years. He was happy there and had no responsibilities and that was how he wanted things to continue.
>
> On Sunday and Wednesday afternoons, visitors would arrive by bus. Contrary to normal practice, the main gates were closed and locked before the arrival of the buses; the visitors would wait until the gates were opened

and they would walk down to the front hall. I imagine staff would accompany them to the appropriate ward to visit their relative. Visiting was, I seem to remember, only 2–4 pm, and certainly only twice a week.

Every weekday morning, the 'hooter' was sounded. This was not an unpleasant sound (unlike the one that took its place after the war) and could be heard on a still day as far as Wallingford. The 8.35 am sounding went on for about 30 seconds and was presumably to let workers know that they were 'on the hurry up' to get to work in time. If the hooter sounded at any other time it was because a patient had absconded. All off-duty staff were expected to turn up at the hospital to find out who was missing and in which direction to search. I never remember anyone being out for too long, unless they had decided to go into the river; this did occasionally happen. My father told me about one patient, completely harmless, but quite an old man, who walked out one day and, search as they might, the staff could not find him. That night there was quite a severe frost and they were all concerned for him but, before the search could resume the following morning, he walked back into the hospital, stark naked. When asked where he had been, he simply said he had been 'out for a night's bleaching'. He didn't get even a cold. They bred them tough in those days.

Until after WW2 there were not many drugs for treating mentally ill patients, so some of the more disturbed people were housed in 'side rooms'. These were rooms off the gallery, which was the long, highly polished ward with chairs along either side. The ward kitchen and dormitory were located either side at the end of the gallery. There were padded rooms where patients who would be likely to harm themselves were housed until they calmed down sufficiently to be back on the ward. Windows were covered with wooden shutters, and someone yelling their head off and banging the shutters was almost my lullaby as a child; certainly, visitors to our house found it a little noisy at times. We didn't notice it. Once the tranquilising drugs were introduced, there was little need for the side rooms, and I believe they were used as bedrooms for the nurses.

Some Anecdotes from the Author's Collection

After some consideration, a few tales from the asylum are offered as impartial illustrations of the real-life struggle between different realities. Consider, if you will, that even what we call normal life often contains events more bizarre than any of these.

During Dr Gilland's tenure, a severely withdrawn and depressed man was, at length, placed in front of a harmonium, which he gradually began to play. As time went on, his evident musical talent was rediscovered, until he was arranging and transcribing music for use by the asylum. On his discharge, Dr Gilland regretted the loss of his very useful abilities.

A male patient persistently hallucinated, seeing pigs' heads appearing out of the ground in front of him as he took his exercise in the courtyard. He kicked at these apparitions and rapidly scuffed out the toes of his boots. Being only human, besides sick and tired of replacing his footwear at frequent intervals, someone judiciously hammered a small nail into the toe of the patient's boot. The next time the patient took a flying kick at the imaginary pigs' heads, he received an early form of aversion therapy. Although this kind of thing was clearly not acceptable, it was apparently quite successful.

A troublesome and destructive female patient in the 1920s had to be confined to a side room and, when needing to use the toilet, would be issued with a rubber chamber pot. On a memorable occasion, someone made a mistake and a china pot was provided. On entering the side room 'post performance', Nurse Lilian Brignall was the unlucky recipient of the flying pot and, worse, its contents. In the 1920s, although nursing staff were issued with winter and summer uniforms, they received only one of each and they did not lend themselves to easy laundering. In consequence, after recovering some of her dignity, Lilian had to wear patients' clothing for the rest of the day.

An unfortunate lady developed a taste for arachnids. She would pop them in her mouth whenever she caught one and later announce to whoever would listen, 'I had a *beautiful* spider today, dear.'

During the mid-1920s, another female patient was in the habit of using a chamber pot, rather than the WCs. Unless the nurses were vigilant, she was liable to stick her head into the pot after making water. Lilian Brignall observed, however, that 'she had the most beautiful head of golden hair'!

A patient called John had charge of the horse-drawn mower that was used to tend the lawns and cricket field. He suffered from religious mania, a recognised psychiatric condition, and one day in the 1930s, to show his devotion he embellished the Oval – that sacrosanct turf inside the carriage circle – with an enormous cross of breadcrumbs. Although his masterpiece was short-lived, one imagines that the local bird population, and perhaps St Francis, were suitably appreciative.

John's other claim to fame was that he was a serial absconder and had, uniquely, taken a graceful flying leap over the ditch surrounding the male airing court and escaped over the wall beyond – which wasn't bad as he was recovering from TB at the time!

There was a classic case of echopraxia, a condition in which the sufferer mimics another person's movements. Two male patients (one of them without the syndrome) would often be seen going about the hospital a few steps apart, so perfectly synchronised in every action that they might have been connected by strings. Neither acknowledged the other's existence. The spectacle fascinated any onlookers and they were known as 'Me and My Shadow'.

One male patient was prepared to take advantage of his station in life. When faced with a long queue for the bus back from Wallingford, he would elbow his way to the front, calling, 'Make way for a Moulsford lunatic!'

Percy Walwyn

It has been the general rule in this account to avoid naming patients but an exception can be justified. Percy Walwyn had apparently been an engineer or draughtsman in professional life and worked for the famous Rudge motorcycle concern. In 1949, following the dawn of the jet age, he produced some intriguing engineering sketches that showed his ideas for swivelling the exhaust of a jet engine as a means of controlling an aeroplane in flight. The drawings were duly consigned to the Air Ministry in London, which pricked up its ears and sent a motorcar full of important people to talk to the inventor at the address neatly inscribed on the sheets. Arriving at the front desk of Fair Mile Hospital, the party was regretfully informed by Leslie Talbot, the Hall Porter, that there was no Mr Percival Walwyn at the hospital – unless they were seeking Percy, who was one of the patients. One can only imagine the feelings of the Air Ministry boffins who, with little further ceremony, turned on their heels and beat a hasty retreat to London.

We may never know for certain whether Percy was a prophet without honour, but it does not appear that anyone else in 1949 had hit upon the principle that came to be known as thrust vectoring and which, much later, made possible the Harrier 'jump-jet'. The principle has since been employed in ways even more closely resembling Walwyn's sketches. In 2009, the author deposited Walwyn's sketches at the National Aerospace Library, Farnborough, Surrey, where they were received with interest and published in the house newsletter.

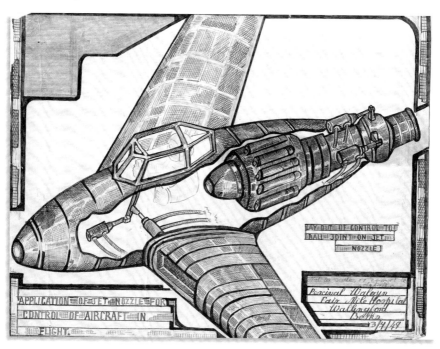

One of Percy Walwyn's far-sighted sketches. (By permission of the Royal Aeronautical Society (National Aerospace Library))

Percy Walwyn's later demise, although tragic, may or may not have been of the saddest kind seen at Fair Mile. He was fond of fishing, which he was allowed to do by the River Thames. A former male nurse related that Percy's eccentric method of casting his fishing line was to whirl around on the spot – to the peril of anyone standing within the compass of rod and line – knowing that centrifugal force would carry float and hook far out into the stream. One day, Percy went missing from the riverside and was later found drowned. No one could tell whether it was accident or suicide.

6

CARE AND TREATMENT

....

I found this institution in excellent order on my visit today. The wards were bright, and well supplied with objects of interest and amusement, and the dormitories were orderly and well ventilated, whilst the bedding throughout was all that could be desired. The gardens associated with the wards, in which there were many patients[26], were well kept, pleasant in appearance and satisfactory in all respects. The general tone of the institution seemed to be one of homely comfort materially contributed to by the good feeling that obviously exists between the patients and the medical and nursing staff.

(Opening paragraph of a report by R.W. Branthwaite, Commissioner of the Board of Control, 1926.)

It is important to set the correct tone on this subject. Despite enduring problems involving buildings, equipment and staffing, there can be no doubt whatsoever that strenuous efforts were always made to make patients' lives safe, comfortable, gainful and free from stress; the sentiments in the above statement were echoed year after year, but sometimes as a prelude to specific criticism.

The craft of psychiatric nursing was in its infancy when the Moulsford Asylum came into being. Psychiatry and its history are subjects far too involved for this book, as is the discovery and development of therapeutic drugs; at the outset, the county asylums had neither. Nor were admissions procedures refined. Although forms had to be completed, Superintendent Douty complained in May 1892, with signs of exasperation, that patients were brought to the asylum by persons unqualified and uninformed in the patient's particulars and circumstances.

Care in the Victorian era was based on a routine of compassion, good hygiene, adequate nourishment and comfort, discipline, work and recreation. This approach, called the Moral Cure by some, was effective in many cases. Gainful employment was held to be an aid to recovery for many patients, who were offered ample opportunity to help in the asylum's gardens, grounds and farm, sewing rooms, workshops, kitchen, laundry and bootmaker's workshop and cleaning the wards. This tradition survived through the transition from 'asylum' to 'hospital' and made good economic sense, as it tended to keep costs down.

Long before the Welfare State, a significant number of patients arrived – sometimes from home but often from the parish workhouses – so stressed by exhaustion, malnutrition or disease that they were vulnerable to mental imbalance and the medical superintendents repeatedly complained about this state of affairs. The situation was exacerbated, around 1875, by a well-intended government subsidy of 4*s* a week per patient. In that year, 43 per cent of Moulsford's admissions were from the workhouses.

Relief from anxiety and deprivation often arrested and reversed patients' decline. Those who improved required less supervision and might progress to supervised activities outside the asylum; records held by the BRO show that up to 40 per cent of patients admitted in the asylum's first five years of operation were able to return home within twelve months.

For some, mental illness owed little to a poor diet, as in the case of diseases that produced psychological side-effects. Again citing the early superintendent's journals at the BRO, there are the examples of tertiary syphilis and post-natal infections – such as puerperal fever – that unbalanced the mind: remedies for these conditions, nowadays preventable or curable with ease, could not be depended on until the advent of penicillin and the advanced drugs of the later twentieth century.

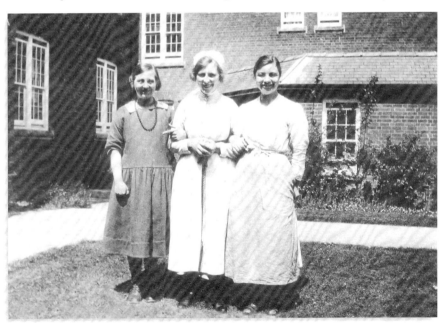

Lilian Brignall (centre) with friends; quite possibly patients. Taken in the airing court next to Female 8 (Ipsden) in 1925. The structure on the right is one of the several external corridors that permitted discreet movement around the hospital. (Vera Wheeler)

TABLE III.—*Showing the Admissions, Discharges, and Deaths, with the mean Annual Mortality and proportion of Recoveries per cent. of the Admissions for each Year since the opening of the Asylum on the 30th September, 1870.*

YEAR	Admitted			Discharged — Recovered			Discharged — Relieved			Discharged — Not Improved			Died			Remaining on 31st of December, each year.			Average numbers resident.			Percentage of Recoveries on Admissions including all transfers.			Percentage of Deaths on average numbers resident.		
	M.	F.	Tot.	M.	F.	Tot.	M.	F.	Tot.	M.	F.	Tot.	M.	F.	Tot.	M.	F.	Tot.	M.	F.	Tot.	M.	F.	Tot.	M.	F.	Tot.
3 Mos. 1870	50	62	112	..	..	..	..	..	..	1	..	1	1	..	1	49	62	111	42	53	95	..	..	..	2·3	..	1·0
1871	85	85	170	4	7	11	3	1	4	..	..	..	13	7	20	116	132	248	80	95	175	4·7	8·2	6·4	16·2	7·3	11·4
1872	40	42	82	19	17	36	4	..	4	3	..	3	14	17	31	124	139	263	120	138	258	40·4	40·4	40·4	11·6	12·3	12·0
1873	35	42	77	13	13	26	1	2	3	8	7	15	14	14	28	123	145	268	129	143	272	37·2	30·9	33·7	10·8	9·0	10·2
1874	42	59	101	7	24	31	..	3	3	4	7	11	23	25	48	127	145	272	122	146	268	25·0	41·0	33·8	18·8	17·1	17·9
1875	32	39	71	8	16	24	4	1	5	2	5	7	18	11	29	130	150	280	128	155	283	25·5	39·2	33·3	14·4	7·0	10·2
1876	43	56	99	11	22	33	..	3	3	4	5	9	12	19	31	145	159	304	134	157	291	27·5	42·5	35·6	8·2	12·1	10·6
1877	43	46	89	15	17	32	4	3	7	16	13	29	14	13	27	139	159	298	148	158	306	25·5	36·9	33·3	9·4	8·2	8·8
1878	40	47	87	11	20	31	2	3	5	6	6	12	14	17	31	146	160	306	145	157	302	27·5	42·5	35·6	9·6	10·8	10·2
1879	40	45	85	20	21	41	1	3	4	3	..	3	22	9	31	140	167	307	143	163	306	50·0	46·7	48·2	15·3	5·5	10·1
1880	86	105	191	17	18	35	..	4	4	6	1	8	16	9	35	192	228	420	157	180	337	15·7	19·0	17·5	10·1	5·5	10·3
1881	46	65	111	17	18	35	..	2	2	2	2	4	23	17	40	196	256	452	196	244	440	36·9	27·6	31·5	11·7	6·9	9·0
1882	70	68	138	13	17	30	4	4	8	1	1	2	29	26	55	222	278	500	201	264	465	18·5	25·0	21·7	14·4	9·8	11·8
1883	46	54	100	17	18	35	2	2	4	1	1	2	28	24	52	218	286	504	221	283	504	36·9	33·3	35·2	12·6	8·4	10·3
1884	45	43	88	19	31	50	6	3	9	21	11	32	31	21	52	190	264	454	204	280	484	42·2	72·0	56·8	15·1	7·5	10·7
1885	45	51	96	15	20	35	3	4	9	2	2	4	16	20	36	196	270	466	200	266	466	33·3	39·2	36·4	8·0	7·5	7·7
1886	45	54	99	6	16	24	9	3	12	2	1	3	16	14	28	214	292	506	207	283	490	17·7	29·6	24·2	6·7	4·9	5·7
1887	53	54	97	11	23	34	6	1	7	2	1	3	36	27	63	209	273	482	207	284	491	20·7	52·3	35·0	17·3	9·5	12·8
1888	43	59	102	12	23	35	1	12	21	1	1	2	27	14	41	209	297	496	210	280	490	27·9	39·0	34·2	12·8	5·0	8·3
1889	37	60	97	8	23	49	5	5	10	1	1	2	9	19	28	212	290	502	214	294	508	48·6	51·6	50·5	4·2	6·4	5·5
1890	43	56	99	11	20	31	3	6	8	5	3	8	20	20	40	218	296	514	218	295	513	25·5	35·7	31·3	9·2	6·7	7·7
1891	48	40	88	13	11	24	1	7	12	3	5	8	22	18	40	218	296	514	225	299	524	27·1	27·5	27·3	9·7	6·0	7·6
1892	49	65	114	19	22	41	2	1	8	8	2	10	14	24	38	226	296	522	234	303	537	38·7	33·8	35·9	5·9	7·9	7·0
1893	44	62	106	14	24	38	3	8	11	3	5	8	18	31	49	234	305	545	237	304	541	31·8	38·7	35·8	7·6	10·2	9·0
1894	60	57	117	14	29	43	2	4	6	2	4	6	19	31	50	240	305	545	247	304	551	23·3	50·8	36·7	7·69	10·19	9·07
1895	52	66	118	23	19	42	1	8	9	5	10	15	25	23	48	257	303	558	252	304	557	44·2	28·6	35·6	9·9	7·5	8·6
1896	49	52	101	20	12	32	4	3	7	2	3	5	23	24	47	255	313	568	255	307	562	40·8	23·0	30·8	9·0	7·8	3·3
	1321	1524	2845	366	511	877	70	102	172	115	94	209	515	504	1019												

NOTE.—The Admissions of 1880 include 92 Patients belonging to Unions in the County of Berks who had previously been maintained in other Asylums, and the Admissions of 1881 include 31 Patients belonging to the County of Surrey.

The percentage of Recoveries upon the Admissions, deducting transfers from other Asylums and from Class to Class, is 39·6 per cent.

Patient statistics for the years 1870 to 1896. (Reproduced by permission of the Berkshire Record Office)

Humane treatment was of paramount concern. The following directive appeared in the opening paragraphs of the 1904 'Regulations and Orders for the Management and Conduct of those engaged in the service of the Berkshire Asylum Wallingford':

> All the patients are held to be not responsible for their words or actions and must be treated with the greatest consideration, sympathy and forbearance by those who are placed in charge of them.

For the sake of space alone, this document will be referred to as the 'Staff Regulations' from this point onwards but the point was well made and the care staff sometimes had to draw on deep reserves of tolerance and forbearance, mixed with amateur psychology, to avoid breaking this cardinal rule.

Nutrition

With bodily health a prerequisite for mental recovery, some detail of the patients' diet (regularly referred to as 'the dietary' in the archives) is appropriate. The author is indebted to a Fair Mile Hospital Newsletter of April 1974 for the following comparison of the dinnertime (that is to say midday) food allowances for patients:

	1870	1903
Sunday	7 oz meat, 4 oz bread, 12 oz potatoes	7 oz meat, 3 oz bread, 12 oz potatoes
Monday	3 oz meat Men: 6 oz bread, 1½ pints soup Women: 4 oz bread, 1 pint soup	3 oz meat, 4 oz bread, 1 oz cheese, 1 pint soup
Tuesday	7 oz meat, 4 oz bread, 12 oz potatoes	6 oz meat, 3 oz bread, 12 oz potatoes
Wednesday	4 oz meat, 12 oz meat-pie	4 oz meat, 12 oz meat-pie
Thursday	7 oz meat, 4 oz bread, 12 oz potatoes	7 oz meat, 3 oz bread, 12 oz potatoes
Friday	4 oz meat, 4 oz bread, 1 pint Irish stew	4 oz meat, 3 oz bread, 1 pint Irish stew
Saturday	4 oz meat	4 oz meat, 3 oz bread, 12 oz potatoes

Occasionally, bacon was substituted for the fresh meat.

At first sight, the fare appears very plain but it represented an adequate and nourishing diet, one that some poorer patients might have found hard to scrape together in life outside. These rations were supplemented by foodstuffs from the farm, kitchen garden and orchard. Given that the asylum also attended to patients' spiritual well-being, it is perhaps surprising to note that fish was not provided on a Friday, but this would have represented a considerable expense.

The newsletter continues:

In addition to this, men and women were each allowed ½ pint beer with their dinner. Breakfast and supper consisted of 6oz bread for men, 5oz for women, together with ⅓oz butter and 1 pint of tea. In 1903, breakfast consisted of 8oz bread for men, 5oz for women with ½oz butter and 1 pint of tea or cocoa.

Patients employed on the land, in workshops and laundry have 2oz bread, 1oz cheese and ½ pint beer at 10 a.m. and 4 p.m. Patients employed in the wards have the same at 10 a.m. only.

In 1903, currant cake was sometimes given instead of bread and butter. On Sundays, 1 gallon tea was made using 1oz tea, 4oz sugar and 1 pint milk. A 1lb plum or suet pudding was made using 8oz flour, 1oz raisins, 1oz treacle and 1oz suet or dripping.

Dr Gilland took an intense interest in the proper nutrition of his charges on a finite budget and in January 1872 expressed satisfaction with trials of New Zealand mutton – possibly shipped canned, since refrigerated shipping from the antipodes was not attempted until 1876. The Steward estimated that mutton-based dishes on three days would require some 120–150lb of meat per week. At Gilland's request, and in line with other asylums, the bread allowance increased in 1875 by 4oz for men and 3oz for women. He commented that the patients 'do not now eat so ravenously as formerly'.

In December 1886, while Dr John Barron was Acting Superintendent, a Mr Hargreaves of Maiden Erlegh donated 100 rabbits to the asylum and was thanked for this notable and welcome change to the menu.

Various aspects of Superintendent J. Harrington Douty's early reports show that he was a man of action and an improver. This 1892 submission to the Visitors shows that he was not only keen to improve the patients' lot, but that he was prepared to go out on a limb to achieve his reasonable ambitions:

Your permission is asked to allow the Superintendent to make an alteration in the Friday's dinner of the patients. This dinner had always been distasteful to a larger number of the patients who on that day constantly go without any dinner rather than partake of it. It consisted of a thin stew or soup made from stale bread collected from the waste of the dining hall, with meat and vegetables. During the summer it was frequently sour and disagreeable owing to the old and sour bread it contained. There was always the difficulty of expense in providing an agreeable substitute. For a few weeks past a stew has been made, which the patients greatly relish and of which they partake heartily. There is the same supply of meat and vegetables with the addition of rice and lump potatoes and the exclusion of the bread. This alteration entails a total increase in the expense of about one third of a penny per head per week. I trust that the Visitors will allow this change to be made permanent as the trifling expense is well spent in providing a more acceptable meal. The yield of potatoes this year is sufficient to meet this extra demand.

It is interesting to note that, in May 1887, several patients were removed to the Reading Union. Superintendent Douty's report of that month recorded his satisfaction that they 'are to receive extra diet at the workhouse'.

Beer is usually a cheerful subject and formed part of the diet of patients and staff alike. In such a large setting, the asylum might have had its own brew house but beer was part of the bought-in provisions and put out to tender. In 1908, the Wallingford Brewery Company quoted for supply of ale at 32*s* per barrel of 36 gallons and beer at 20*s* per barrel of 36 gallons. Both offers were accepted and the author craves the reader's indulgence while he considers the current price of these beverages and wipes a small tear from his eye.

Beer, incidentally, was part of the allowances to staff, listed as 'emoluments' to their wage or salary until 1910, when a monetary allowance was substituted. In the days before treated mains water, drinking beer (often weak 'small beer') was a way of avoiding waterborne infections and it was commonly supplied to labourers and servants.

It can generally be said that care and forethought, sometimes modified by experience, went into feeding the patients. The Commissioners in Lunacy had high but realistic standards and recorded adjustments and improvements over the years – not always approving of what they saw, as in their April 1924 comment that patients appeared generally well nourished, but that 'this was not previously always the case'. Commissioner Rollisham noted in 1925 that 'The diet has been improved considerably over the past few years and still greater variety will be given when new cooking apparatus has been added to the kitchen plant', while his colleagues Bailey and Branthwaite said in January 1926 that they were 'especially pleased with the care taken to provide an adequate amount of fresh vegetables and fruit'.

If it's Stew, it Must be Friday

Repetition and predictability in the dining hall had become an issue by 1932, when moves to re-sequence the dinner menu, advocated in several previous years, were considered overdue. This was finally achieved in time for the 1937 inspection!

Fish, not previously seen on the menu, became available with the arrival of a fish fryer late in 1934, although ready-made fishcakes were to be served, rather than fresh fish. The same Commissioners' report observed:

> Today's dinner consisted of boiled heart and two vegetables & looked appetising but examining into the diet we came to the conclusion that it might be on a more generous scale and we discussed various methods of improving it with Dr Holder (Deputy Medical Superintendent).

July 1936, on the other hand, brought news that:

> The patients' diet is varied and generous & a particularly important and valuable feature is the ample supply of green vegetables and fresh fruit, grown on the estate. We understand that almost all the jams consumed by the patients are made on the premises from home-grown fruit.

The 1939 Commissioners' report mentioned that dinners could be quite cold on arrival in the wards but, allowing for the fact that an inspector's job is to keep an organisation on its toes, the temperature of meals was by this time less of an issue than the parlous state of the kitchen itself, related in Chapter 3. Some details of wartime catering issues are discussed in Chapter 7.

Comfort and Security

Most wards consisted of a 'gallery' or wide corridor with ample seating and daylight, which connected to a day room with tables and chairs. Doors along one side of the gallery led to offices, nurses' sleeping accommodation, a ward kitchen and 'side rooms' for more disruptive patients. From some of the earliest photographs available, it is clear that the patients' accommodations were designed to be comfortable

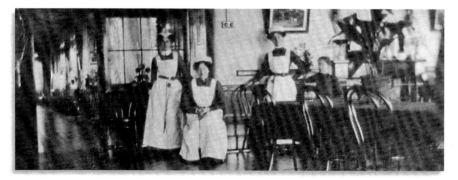

This is thought to be Female 7 (later Goring) ward at Christmas 1913. This is the day room, with the gallery beyond. (Spackman collection)

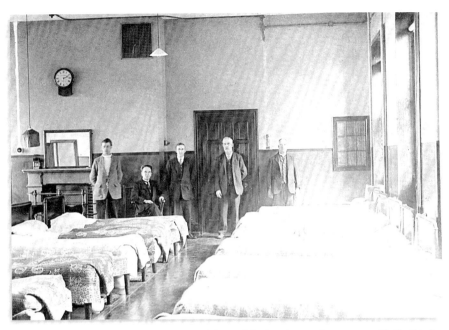

The dormitory of Male 4 in about 1919. It is possible that the gentleman seated is Dr Edwin
Lindsay Dunn, Superintendent from 1918 to 1920. (Spackman collection)

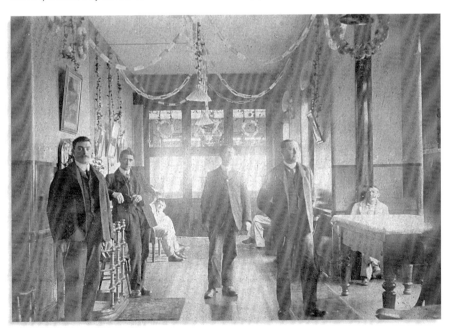

Taken from a used postcard, this is Christmas 1913 in a Male ward. The man on the left is
Will Bunning, Charge Attendant, who wrote to his mother explaining that his short jacket
was the result of a shortage of cloth. Will served from 1904 to 1938. The other men standing
are probably doctors or senior officers. (Spackman collection)

although some of the interior features, such as panelling in the galleries, were added as part of Hine's *c.*1900 alterations. Although dormitories were the norm throughout the life of the hospital, they were at least spacious and properly furnished, with high ceilings and plenty of window area.

Considerable trouble was taken to add homely touches to the wards, such as pictures on the walls, flowers from the hospital gardens, magazines, books and indoor games (such as bagatelle, draughts, Ludo and billiards), even pianos. Whilst the standard of decoration and home comforts was liable to vary over the years, the prevailing attitude was that some semblance of home life had to be provided.

It is no secret that padded rooms were a feature of asylum life and there were occasions when patients had to be confined for their own safety or that of others. However, this was uncommon and precise routines and records had to be kept if a padded room or other form of restraint was used. Also, an attendant was always present, usually outside the open door unless the patient was particularly violent. The Commissioners would comment favourably if there had been no cause to use either 'seclusion' or restraint. These were generally a last resort since sedatives – albeit primitive opiates such as laudanum, or paraldehyde – were often helpful.

It is not pleasant to contemplate steel bars in a mental hospital but a number of iron gates were fitted in the corridors in 1923. The reason was entirely based on the occupants' comfort, since the gates permitted otherwise locked doors to remain open, affording much better circulation of air in hot weather.

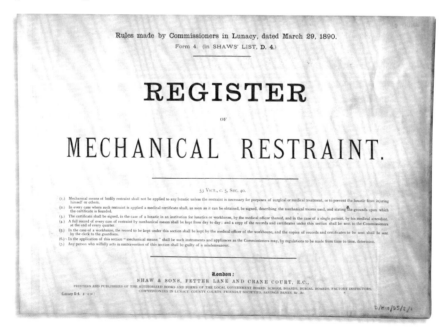

Restraint being regarded as a last resort, all instances had to be recorded in this register. (Reproduced by permission of the Berkshire Record Office)

Hygiene

Early records mention the 'lime-whiting' or whitewashing of the ward walls – usually because it was overdue. Whitewash has deodorant properties and Dr Gilland evidently thought it an aid to health.

From the outset, baths and hot water were provided – at least while Haden's heating system was behaving itself – and patients were bathed weekly unless otherwise required. Two baths could sometimes be found in a single bathroom, a state of affairs picked up by the Commissioners as late as 1933, who recommended a screen or curtain for the sake of patients' dignity. Hair was to be kept clean and brushed. Male patients were shaved twice a week and their hair cut monthly. Men could cultivate their facial hair, provided that the results were tidy; however, no patient was ever allowed to touch either razor or sharp scissors, for fear of disastrous consequences.

Given these words that, in January 1912, flowed from the collective pen of the Commissioners for Lunacy following a tour of inspection, it is impossible not to mention something as fundamental as toilet paper in the context of patient wellbeing:

> In the interest of cleanliness, the absence of any soft toilet requisites[27] such as are now almost invariably used in asylums is to be regretted.

The informed response from the Visitors, besides advocating thrift, was in some ways positively visionary:

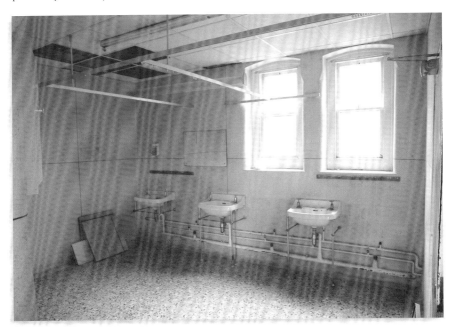

One of the communal washrooms that survived up to closure. (Bill Nicholls)

As the cost of this innovation would be very considerable – about £50 per annum, without any apparent benefit to the patients – we do not see our way to recommend the substitution. There would be great waste from misuse by the patients and the constant temptation to place the rolls of paper down the W.C. pans and block the traps. There has been no anal disease from the use of the ordinary newspaper.

Perhaps, by 11 April 1924, Commissioner R.H. Trevor had recovered from this rebuff when he observed, 'I notice that only newspaper is supplied in the W.C.s: an uncomfortable practice now obsolete.'

Returning to January 1912, it was recorded that some poorly enamelled washbasins installed in the 1881 extensions were unsightly and unsanitary. Ever thrifty, the Visitors' response – astonishing to modern sensibilities – was to have the remaining white enamel removed from the metal basins and to continue using them. However, expenditure was authorised in March to replace some badly rusted examples in the Female hospital with modern equipment from the well-known firm of Doulton & Sons. The relatively mundane saga of substandard washbasins, and the 'sanitary annexes' in which they were situated, dragged on until well after the Second World War and contributes to the impression that the hospital suffered from lengthy periods when either money, clear direction or initiative were in short supply.

Dentistry

This subject receives little mention. Surprisingly, a March 1925 report by Commissioner Rollisham tells us 'it was unsatisfactory to find that neither tooth or nail brushes are issued to the wards for the use of any patients who desire to have them'. The July 1948 report brought the good news that 'A room has been fitted up as a dental surgery adjacent to the Laundry Ward', balanced by this slightly barbed observation:

At present the dentist attends on one half day each fortnight only. We think however that the former weekly sessions should be re-introduced, and until the arrears are overtaken even more frequent visits are desirable.

Physical Disease

The physical wellbeing of patients was quite as important as their mental condition and this consideration extended to the nursing staff, who were vulnerable to dangerous diseases in this densely populated and closed environment.

On 19 November 1886, Acting Superintendent Barron reported that, since the heating had been turned on for winter, there had been outbreaks of unusual illnesses including erysipelas (a severe and potentially fatal skin infection that can follow 'strep throat' or an infected wound). Sufferers were confined to the isolation hospital[28] and, in December, Barron saw that they were on the mend. A further five cases developed the next January, when very cold weather again confined patients to the wards. Although they were again cured, there is no record of the treatment actually used: nothing as convenient or effective as penicillin existed at that time.

March 1887 saw the first monthly report of Superintendent J. Harrington Douty, who noted that both the Male and Female hospitals (meaning the infirmary wards) were very full, but with what he considered to be unextraordinary cases, 'chiefly pneumonic' and calling for no special notice. But he also had to record the death from pneumonia of male attendant Philip Hardy, who had probably been infected in the course of his work. The unfortunate Hardy was buried in Cholsey churchyard and his colleagues subscribed a total of £8 to purchase a headstone.

Influenza was a danger to a closed community like the BMH, especially in the lethal 1918–20 pandemic. Happily, outbreaks were usually short-lived and without fatalities. Perhaps more worrying were the likes of scarlet fever and diphtheria. In June 1887, Douty had to cope with an outbreak of scarlet fever and succeeded in isolating it in Female 8. Nevertheless, additional staffing was needed, which stretched the system to its limit. As his staff responded well, he requested handsome gratuities of 10s for both of the volunteer nurses who assisted in the isolation ward. Another outbreak in 1909 was introduced on a doll, brought by family members as a gift to an 11-year-old asylum patient. En route, the family had visited a baby with the disease, who must have handled the doll.

A 1939 report tells us that, owing to a diphtheria outbreak that had lasted all year and affected nurses, Schick testing had been carried out and 'positives' immunised, but that throat and nasal swabbing was impossible in the continued absence of a pathology laboratory. Testing was still not regularly available at the hospital, being carried out either in Reading or Oxford.

Taking a random example, the Commissioners found that, of 779 patients resident in October 1923, only sixty-six were in bed: thirty-four receiving psychiatric treatment; twenty with senile debility and twelve for 'ordinary sickness … a condition that speaks well for the general health of the institution, which seemed to me very good.'

Thankfully, smallpox does not seem to have affected the hospital.

Medicinal Alcohol

Sensitive readers, already reeling from the above-mentioned account of beer prices, may wish to brace themselves before learning that August 1887 brought an initiative from Superintendent Douty to reduce the asylum's outlay on spirituous liquors for medicinal purposes. He asked the Visitors if he might be allowed to administer Scotch whiskey at 19s per gallon, instead of brandy at 24s per gallon!

Enteric Diseases

Typhoid, diarrhoea, enteric fever and dysentery cropped up periodically, sometimes confined to particular areas, sometimes widespread. At various times from 1874, well and borehole water was tested and found blameless, although a shallow well was condemned in 1889. Faults in the drains, soil pipes, water closets, etc. were repaired. Suspicion then fell on the sewage beds – especially when relatively close to the affected parts of the hospital – and only farmyard dung was to be used for gardens, while vegetable growing in the sewage-fed gardens was banned for three years with no benefit. New sewage beds were created close to the river by Messrs Bailey & Denton, sanitary engineers. Disease 'carriers' were implicated and floors lifted to disinfect the soil beneath, but staff members as well as patients suffered and died. Other asylums were also affected, although not as badly as the Berkshire Lunatic Asylum. Laundry practices may have been partly responsible, as related in Chapter 3.

Enteric diseases remained a worry. The BRO holds a lengthy report that relates outbreaks of enteric diseases to the asylum's sanitary arrangements and extensive measures to prevent infection. There was a trouble-free period in the 1920s and 1930s, followed by a series of outbreaks beginning with paratyphoid fever in September 1941. The water and milk were scrutinised 'but neither … is likely to be the source of the present infection, as the outbreak is confined to one female ward, Ward 6'. Immunisation was undertaken, plus a search for carriers in Female 6 and the kitchens. Meanwhile, all drinking water was boiled. The outbreak lasted through the autumn and re-appeared in April 1942, spreading to the Male side with a total of thirteen cases. Meanwhile, Sonne dysentery appeared in March 1942 and spread from Female to Male, totalling forty cases. The outbreaks were brought under control soon after.

Two active carriers of typhoid were found in Male 4 in 1944 but precautions proved effective and just one case in 1945 caused all the staff and admissions patients to be inoculated.

After a trouble-free interval, 103 male and 338 female cases of dysentery ruined the winter of 1947–48. Sulpha drugs were administered and only two cases remained as the NHS era dawned in July 1948. The outbreak was traced to a male carrier who had been cleaning kitchen utensils. The entire hospital population was screened via the Public Health Laboratory in Oxford.

Tuberculosis was present from the asylum's earliest days and there seemed always to be at least a few cases – often more per capita than in comparable institutions. Although commendable figures were achieved through the 1920s and 1930s (10 cases in nineteen months, recorded in 1923), 1942 saw 12 cases per 1,000 against the national average of 11.3, although the death rate of 8 per 1,000 was below the national figure of 8.7. There were twelve deaths in the reporting period. This revived an apparently endless campaign to acquire X-ray equipment and verandahs where patients could be treated in the fresh air (see page 103):

The Public Health Service of Oxford under Professor Wilson continues to render very important aid to the hospital in dealing with its infectious diseases. It is hoped that in the near future micro-radiography for the early diagnosis of pulmonary tuberculosis may become available; meanwhile chest radiography is done at the Royal Berkshire Hospital, and the examination of sputum is carried out in the small pathological laboratory … made by the adaptation of a staff bedroom off Male 2 ward.

The disease remained troublesome, increasing as the hospital came under NHS control. The County TB Officer was a frequent visitor but there was neither X-ray equipment nor chest physician until 1950. The Bungalow was again in use as a TB sanatorium in 1957.

Fresh Air

The beneficial effects of fresh air, notably for cases of tuberculosis – or phthisis, as it was then known – were understood and had frequently been advocated since about 1912. The absence of verandahs was a sore point for decades, starting in that year, when the Visitors and medical staff hoped that open-air treatment could commence; there were plans for a lean-to shelter alongside the external corridor serving Female 8 but none for the Male side. That July, a shelter was approved by 5 votes

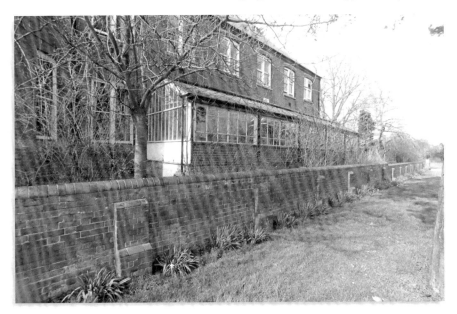

The long-awaited *c*.1930 verandah on the rear of Male 8 (Hermitage) ward. This and an equivalent on Female 8 (Ipsden) are clearly shown on a 1936 Ordnance Survey map. (Spackman collection)

to 3 but a glass roof over it was rejected by 5 votes to 4, sanctioning only a slate one. It was November before the Lunacy Commissioners themselves authorised an outdoor shelter in the Female airing court, but even this was deferred for six months and never materialised.

April 1924 dawned with the lament, 'There are no verandahs or other facilities for nursing suitable cases in the open air.' Prevarication finally gave way to stern demands by the end of 1927, when Female 8 dormitory at last acquired a balcony on its south-east side. Harking back to earlier reluctance to spend money on doing the job properly, the Commissioners observed: 'When a glazed roof is added, it will make an excellent verandah.' The imminent arrival of an equivalent on Male 8 in May 1929 (first reported as being in use in March 1931) suggests that the investment proved worthwhile. However, the subject recurred in 1947 and 1948, when there were twenty cases of TB crowded into the 'F6 sick dormitory' for want of a verandah, and again in 1954 when there was apparently still no Female verandah.[29]

Interventional Psychiatric Therapy

A history of its development is not in the scope of this book but, in the simplest terms, interventional treatment – as distinct from mere sedation – required facilities, skilled personnel and, when appropriate, specialised drugs.

In 1926 there was mention of eleven deaths from general paralysis (neurosyphilis) and a query as to whether arrangements could not be made for 'pyrescial' (fever-related) treatment of this disease at a suitably equipped hospital, by the proven method of induced malaria. General paralysis, schizophrenia and depression could be relieved by infecting the patient with the malaria parasite or, from about 1930, by means of cardiazol shock or insulin coma therapy, which induced convulsions and coma. The procedures were not without risk but were undertaken at the BMH. By 1939, three doctors supported the superintendent in such matters but they still lacked a treatment area; consequently these alarming treatments might be administered in the wards, albeit behind screens.

'Electric shock treatment still gives satisfaction for cases of depression, but cardiazol is favoured for the treatment of schizophrenia. Epanation (meaning trephination or trepanning) is proving satisfactory in the treatment of epilepsy.' (1941)

Electro-convulsive Therapy

Appearing in about 1940, electro-convulsive therapy (ECT) was considered less traumatic and more convenient, although it was still used alongside modified insulin shock therapy in at least 1947. The patient's convulsions could result in broken bones and ECT's reputation flagged until new muscle relaxants and sedatives were available to prevent injuries. It remains in use but has largely been supplanted by effective drugs.

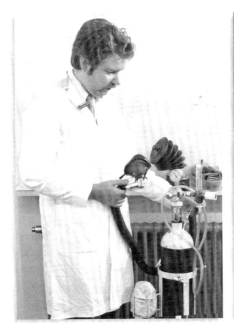

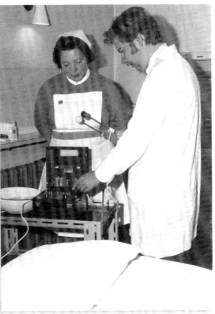

Student Nurse Einar Haukland works in the ECT Treatment Clinic of the George Schuster Hospital. (Spackman collection)

Carmel Parkinson and Einar Haukland preparing ECT equipment in the Schuster in 1972. (Spackman collection)

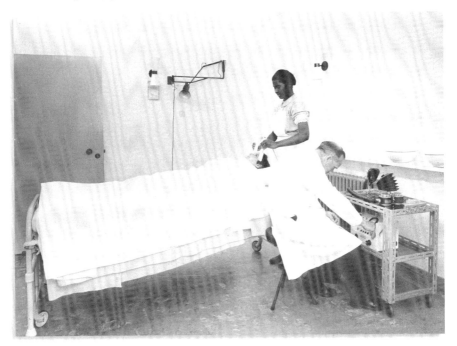

A posed illustration of ECT in the early 1960s, taken in the George Schuster Hospital. (Spackman collection)

Brain Surgery

No information has been found about trephination at the BMH, except that it was thought to be effective for epilepsy. From 1948, some surgical procedures were carried out in the new operating theatre, including pre-frontal lobotomy (leucotomy). More complex procedures were still carried out at the Royal Berkshire Hospital or the Oxford's Radcliffe Infirmary. Although often successful, direct brain surgery carried risks of serious collateral damage and this procedure was also largely superseded by drugs. The last operation was carried out in about 1955, after which the theatre was adapted for other uses.

Therapeutic Drugs

This account cannot do justice to the development of drugs that were of value in psychiatric disease. Little enough was available around 1900, other than sedatives such as bromides, laudanum, morphine, hyoscine, chloral hydrate and paraldehyde. The early barbiturates appeared from 1904, serving as sedatives and anticonvulsants. Chlorpromazine (Largactil), an anti-psychotic, made an enormous impact in the 1950s, along with phenobarbitol, a barbiturate anti-convulsant. By 1960 the Commissioners were able to observe the striking tranquillity of the patients, not least because diazepam (Valium) and antidepressants had further advanced the

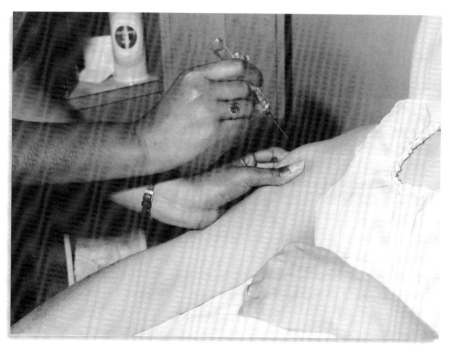

In this posed shot, the injection is administered by Momena Wright, who later held a senior administrative position. (Spackman collection)

cause of cure as opposed to containment. Such progress reduced the pressure on hospital accommodation and facilitated 'care in the community' approaches. There are those who remain unconvinced that this is a valid strategy but at least the spectre of long-term confinement is thankfully fading as medication hastens the demise of the traditional mental hospital.

Readers may care to look up an excellent account of earlier treatment methods, compiled by Epsom & Ewell History Explorer, which at the time of writing can be found at www.ezitis.myzen.co.uk/briefhistorytreatments.html.

7

TWO
WORLD WARS

....

The traumatic events of 1914–18 and 1939–45 influenced the fortunes and func-
tioning of the BMH, although not always directly; shell-shocked and traumatised
servicemen, for example, do not seem to have figured large in the story. More to the
point were the knock-on effects of military requirements, shortages and the inevitable shifts in the nation's scale of priorities.

Specific information from the Great War period is scarce, especially while patient
records remain closed. The BRO does, however, inform us that a number of the
nation's asylums were taken over for military use, displacing large numbers of
patients to other facilities. We hear that the Sussex County Asylum had to transfer
patients to the BMH, which also took in a small number of German prisoners of
war, although it otherwise saw little change in its fortunes except in staffing. Over
the decades, many of the superintendents' monthly reports highlight the endemic
problem of finding enough competent care staff, but male attendants going away to
war caused particular concern. Despite rising patient numbers, days of form-filling
and every legitimate manoeuvre – including attending local military tribunals in
pursuit of exemptions – Superintendent Murdoch was unable to prevent his male
contingent being whittled down from thirty-eight to twenty-four by 1916.

The Second World War saw these patterns repeated, with clear records of patients
moving in from Hill End Hospital in St Albans and Brookwood Hospital in Woking,
Surrey, both having been taken over as Emergency Medical Service hospitals. Hill End
added 300 to the BMH's patient numbers in November 1939, leading to serious overcrowding, the worst aspect being a surplus of 200 on the Female side during the day.
Efforts were made to board out some patients, usually at Hungerford Public Assistance
Institution (the former Poor Law Institute or workhouse, where this practice had been
going on since about 1929), but the move was delayed while a reconstruction scheme
at Hungerford remained unfinished. The year 1940 saw a further influx of seventy
servicemen[30] from the Royal Naval Hospital at Great Yarmouth, Norfolk, by which
time seventy-two men and forty-eight women had been found accommodation at
Hungerford. The ex-Brookwood intake of 100 women arrived in 1941, moving into
Male wards 2 and 3 and necessitating the division of the Villa into two wards.

The war undoubtedly saw the hospital's peak number of patients but the 'headline' maximum is not altogether clear, as the statistics are a little fragmentary and open to interpretation. The highest number in residence that is readily apparent from the Commissioners' annual reports is the 1,274 of the year 1939. By 1942, those in residence were recorded as just 1,154 but, by adding sixty-five absent on leave or trial release, plus 138 boarded out, the total of 1,357 at least approaches the figure of 1,400 claimed by the BRO.

On the staffing front, the Second World War was characterised by the seemingly hopeless task of finding enough nurses. Whilst men were few enough as a result of being called up or taking other war work (even being recalled to the mines), the shortage of women became nothing less than critical. At the outbreak of war, the hospital had sixty male nurses and sixty-four female, the latter already twenty-two under strength. To make matters worse, although their competence was not questioned, most had yet to qualify. In 1941, female nurses numbered just fifty-three, although there was a recovery after that before a post-war decline described by the Commissioners as 'very grave'.

AIR RAIDS AND MOTHERLY LOVE

Being a large target, there was understandable concern that the BMH would be bombed. Give or take a trailer pump for the hospital's fire brigade, air-raid precautions were considered adequate in 1940 and only one incident received much attention.

The first air-raid warning occurred in the early morning of 4 September 1940, whereupon Lilian Talbot hurried her daughter and son away from the hospital to Bow Bridge, a quiet place close to the Thames. Nothing whatever happened and, after enjoying the sights and sounds of serene nature until the 'all clear' sounded, they went home.

One night not long after, perhaps early in 1941, a German bomber dropped a 'stick' of bombs in a long line that cut across the roads linking Cholsey with Wallingford. The bombs penetrated deep into marshy ground and didn't go off. When all this was discovered, both roads were closed as a precaution and Vera and John Talbot, who had meanwhile gone to school in Wallingford, were effectively stuck there. Lilian bravely cycled forth to deliver money so that they could return on the branch-line train. Halted at the roadblock, she remonstrated with the policeman in charge and made it quite clear that she was going along the road to Wallingford no matter what. She was allowed to proceed at her own risk and later said that she had never pedalled so fast in her life!

It soon became clear that some of the bombs had fallen almost exactly where the Talbots had taken shelter in September and many believe they are still down there somewhere.

The wartime shortage of men meant that women took secretarial and clerical positions that were previously male preserves. In 1942, Dr Sylvia Reid was temporarily assisting Dr Astley Cooper and from 1945 a female doctor joined the permanent staff for the first time.

Supplies and Rationing

Fears of a German invasion were real enough that, in 1941, supplies such as bags of cereals and a 'rescue' drug supply were dispersed to some old cellars near the main store in case of enemy attack, with other such measures under consideration.

Also in 1941, with rationing in force, some bright spark came up with the idea – as practiced in other hospitals – of putting a supply of sugar on the wards for use in 'hot beverages' by those who took it. Although this seems blindingly obvious, it was actually to save sugar since tea was always made in bulk, ready-sweetened regardless of patients' preferences.

Rationing affected the hospital as it did the civilian population. Despite this, official observations of the patients' diet remained favourable, although it is tempting to suppose that special efforts would have been made to coincide with the dates of the Commissioners' inspections. There were several expressions of approval at the varied nature of the meal planning and efforts to avoid predictability.

From 22 October 1942:

> With the exception of cheese, bacon and eggs, the full civilian ration of rationed foods is issued, and full use is made of the available 'points'. Cheese, bacon and eggs are however very important articles of diet, and we strongly urge that the present issue (1 to 2oz bacon, 3oz cheese – working patients get the full ration – and no eggs) should be brought up to the amount of the full civilian ration. The daily issue of milk a head to patients on ordinary diet is very small, ¼ pint, and every effort should be made to increase this. The allowance of milk for staff is ½ pint daily.

Vera Wheeler recalls that, perhaps due to ministry control, there were no chickens at the hospital during the war, which might explain the absence of eggs. But, considering that the BMH had its own dairy herd, the Commissioners had previously made a slightly surprising comment in 1939 when it observed that the supply of 56 gallons of fresh milk per day was too little for 1,203 patients[31] (it works out to just over ⅓ pint) and that too much use was made of condensed milk. By late 1940, the milk supply had been augmented but there was the surprise discovery that there was no milk cooler in the dairy.

July 1943 brought guarded optimism:

Recently a statistical analysis has been made of the patients' dietary at this
hospital. We were glad to find that no time has been lost in rectifying the deficiencies indicated by this analysis. The issue in bulk of food stuffs with the
right proportion of various ingredients does not necessarily ensure that each
meal is satisfactory.

The patients' dinner yesterday consisted of fish-cakes (containing much
potato), potatoes, haricot beans and a baked sponge pudding sweetened with
jam. It did not appear to us to be a well-balanced meal. Doubtless the uncertain delivery of food-stuffs at the time they are required render catering very
difficult at present: but we hope this aspect of the dietary will be kept in mind
in the planning of each day's meals.

Also:

We discussed with the Medical Superintendent and the Clerk and Steward
the desirability of giving supper to all patients. At present only a few of the
male workers have this meal. The chief difficulty arises from the nurses' hours
of duty and whilst the present scarcity of nurses lasts, there is no prospect of
reorganising their duties.

Regardless of staff shortages, and while such concern is clearly laudable, it is hard to
see how this could be achieved with rationing the way it was.

Natural Instincts

With the country crammed with men in uniform, a hospital full of young nurses was
like a magnet to servicemen from nearby RAF Benson and the American airfield at
Mount Farm (Berinsfield). They were barred from the hospital grounds but waited
en masse at the main gate, vying to attract a nurse's favour, while the girls always
dressed up to look their best. Some of the romantic antics that took place at the
end of the evening on the same spot – or, indeed, illicitly inside the grounds – are
better not related, but were long imprinted on the memories of the family living at
the Lodge.

8

OCCUPATIONAL THERAPY AND WORK THERAPY

· ·

The asylum's Victorian ethos put much emphasis on providing the patients with useful occupations, to give their lives form and purpose and a measure of self-respect. Many of these have already been mentioned.

In January 1930, referring to the success seen in other hospitals, Commissioner Rollisham proposed the appointment of 'a female occupation officer whose duty would be to teach and interest those patients who now sit about all day doing nothing'.

The Commissioners' report of 1931 makes the earliest known recommendation of 'occupation therapy' (OT), although nothing had been put in place up to that time. The following year, we hear that Dr Read had proposed an OT room in the Bungalow, although nothing indicates that this came to pass. At the same time, some women were said to be doing OT and it was thought that men might soon join in. By 1933, despite the Commissioners' continued advocacy, only modest progress had been made, with nine or ten men working on rug making, fretwork and raffia work. It was suggested that the Matron and Head Male Nurse visit one or two hospitals where such a programme was valued!

With the impending opening of the Villa, 1935 saw the Commissioners hoping 'that opportunity will be taken to develop occupations in this building, which would encourage an atmosphere of interest and activity'. Suffice to say that this aspiration was not fulfilled but the report was able to add:

In the wards of the main building & elsewhere we saw some attractive embroidery and were glad to hear that competitions are held and prizes given. For the men, the room mentioned at last visit is in use, for about 12 patients, who do rug making, envelope making and one or two other handicrafts, but there is still scope for extension in the wards.

The story was much the same in 1936, although tinged with optimism:

… there is still scope for extension of this form of activity. Such articles as rugs, coat hangers, fretwork etc. are made in the wards and many of them are of good design and finish. In the sewing room, such of the female patients as are able are allowed to make their own frocks, a privilege which we are quite sure is much appreciated.

Yet by December 1938, OT had still not been formally established, leading to suggestions that nurses obtain some knowledge of the subject. Mrs Astley Cooper, wife of the new superintendent, was meanwhile leading sessions on three days weekly. Working in the divided sewing room, the good lady struggled valiantly through 1939 but lacked trained assistance. As a result, many patients sat around doing nothing.

Finally, in 1940, a Miss Taylor was appointed Occupational Therapist. Both Male and Female sides were covered and she had plans to expand the scope of OT, starting with the Male side which, by the end of 1941, offered basket weaving, reed weaving, cabinet work and joinery. The war hampered her work, as it did many aspects of the hospital's activities, but late 1942 saw her coping with 100-plus women and twenty men; however, there remained an unhelpful lack of enthusiasm for the function in the wards.

The term *occupational* therapy first appears in July 1943, at which time classes were held daily for fifty-two women and eighteen men. The repeated call for extra space for this function had gone unanswered for yet another year.

The Commissioners commented in 1943:

> Large groups of patients are employed in the utility departments – sewing room, laundry, kitchen and gardens more especially. Some of the male workers have liberal issues of tobacco, but no corresponding inducement is given to the women workers. We hope the Committee will give further consideration to the issuing of tokens that can be exchanged for articles, tobacco or sweets at the Canteen – a department that continues to function actively in spite of war-time restrictions.

This is an interesting observation on the unequal treatment sometimes meted out to women and on the general principle that effort should be rewarded. Happily, women were given cigarettes for their efforts from 1944.

The remaining war years saw little change in circumstances or the numbers of patients using OT, although records indicate that larger accommodation was eventually found for the men. The OT room was still within the hospital and almost certainly in part of the women's sewing room.

Starting her training at the BMH in 1921, Lilian Brignall won her RMN[32], left the hospital's employ in 1926 to marry Hall Porter Leslie Talbot and, by 1949, had raised two children in the Lodge. She then retrained and returned to what was now Fair Mile in the role of Occupational Therapist. She was a capable, no-nonsense woman, daughter of Stoker Ernest Brignall, and her upbringing in a large village family, followed by a period in domestic service, had equipped her with a range of practical skills. She put these to good use, teaching sewing, knitting, weaving, embroidery, rug-making and cane work to her female charges. Male patients, usually supervised by male staff, were offered some of these options but could also do carpentry, printing, basket making and other 'male-orientated' crafts.

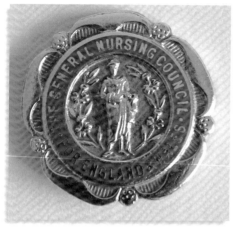

Lilian Brignall's RMN badge. (David Talbot)

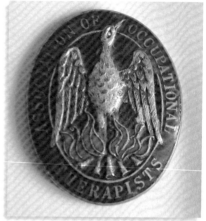

Lilian Talbot's Association of Occupational Therapists badge. (David Talbot)

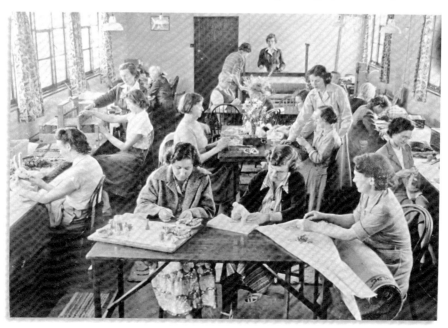

A posed but busy scene in Female Occupational Therapy in about 1957. Patients are sewing, weaving and making rugs and soft toys. The lady seated left at the nearest table appears to be painting plaster of Paris figures. Mrs Talbot (standing, left) presides, with Pamela Bunker at the far end of the room. (Spackman collection)

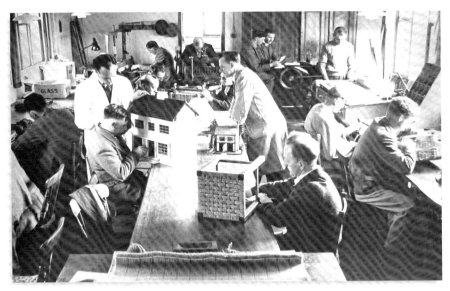

Male patients busy in their OT hut in about 1957. The man leaning on the table is Taff Jones, Charge Nurse. (Spackman collection)

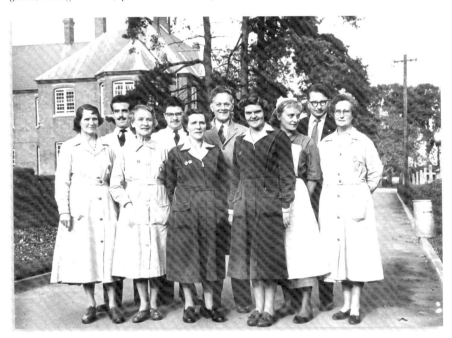

Occupational therapy staff and nurses outside the OT huts in October 1958. From left: Mrs Lambert; Francisco 'Frank' Plazas (Spanish); Vi Perry; Albert Kennedy; Lilian Talbot; 'Taff' Jones; Joyce Sherwood; Colette Dusaillent (French); Michael Truba (Latvian); Beatrice West. Male 8 (Hermitage) ward is behind on the ground floor, with 9 (Ilsley) ward above. Frank Plazas came to Fair Mile in 1956 and is father of opera star Mary Plazas. He was assigned to OT when this photo was taken. (Frank Plazas)

From 1950, OT was based in two wooden huts[33] – one Male, one Female –
beyond the service road at the rear of the Victorian buildings, a stone's throw from
the Recreation Hall. The unit had two qualified female therapists, backed up by OT
assistants and assigned student nurses. In the group photo of 1958, two of the four
men are students from the overseas intakes that followed the war.

An impressive range of craft items was produced by OT in the 1950s under
Mrs Talbot's guidance. Soft toys were a particular speciality, alongside artificial
flowers (in these pre-plastic days, artfully constructed from wire and dyed nylon
stockings), lampshades, plaster figurines, dolls' houses, model boats, baskets and
stools, many of which did yeoman service in local households.

Lilian retired in 1962. A matter of a year or so later, the nature of occupational
therapy changed significantly, especially with the advent of the new Work Therapy
building, where OT relocated, and craft-based activities gave way to unskilled tasks,
such as clipping together plastic toys. These were supposed to generate an income
for the patients, although the rate was small. Needless to say, given her range of
abilities, Lilian had a pretty low opinion of this turn of events.

By the end of the twentieth century, OT was again teaching creative skills and
facilities: a number of fashionable activities such as potting, batik, music and computing were on offer, assisted by well-qualified staff.

Work therapy, as an identified discipline, appears to be a distinctly post-war arrival.
The activities seem to have centred around 'outsourced' tasks under Remploy or
similar organisations. A rather unnerving undertaking of 1957 was the manufacture

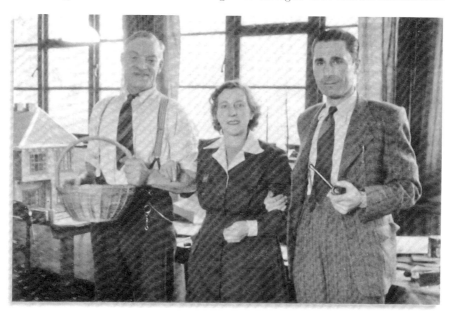

George Herring (left), an accomplished basket maker, with Lilian Talbot in about 1950.
(Vera Wheeler)

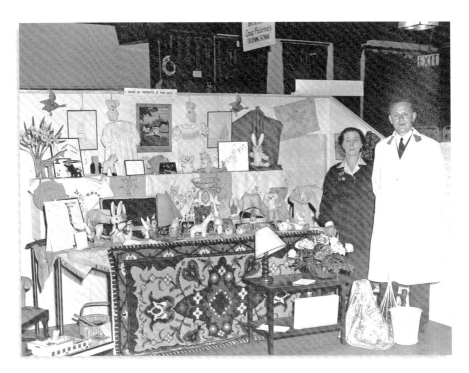

Occupational Therapy handicrafts on display about 1955. The venue may be Reading Town Hall. Lilian Talbot and Taff Jones are presiding. (Author's collection)

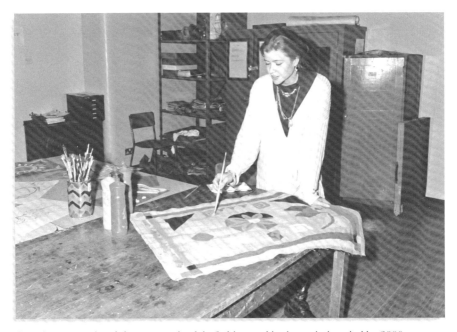

Creative occupational therapy was back in fashion and in the main hospital by 2000. Occupational Therapist Sarah Childs demonstrates. (Spackman collection)

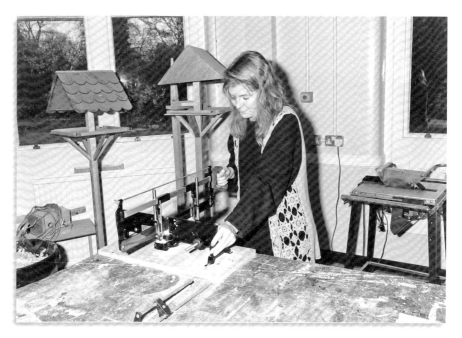

Practical skills were also taught in the closing years of Fair Mile. (Spackman collection)

of fireworks, by both men and women, in the cricket pavilion. The pavilion survived – perhaps because the scheme did not run for very long. In 1960, we are told that only men were involved in work therapy, although this may refer to the accommodation then available; the need for a dedicated space had been pointed out. In that year, old telephones were being dismantled for their parts.

We will leave the subject with a story that may be apocryphal but which still has its supporters. At the time when there was an embargo on imports from South Africa, tinned fruit from that country was supposedly brought to Fair Mile to be re-labelled as Rhodesian. The tale has been strenuously denied but, whether true or not, makes an interesting commentary on the general character of work therapy in what was, perhaps, an isolated 'dark' period.

9

SOCIAL ACTIVITIES
AND RECREATION

From the asylum's earliest years, the authorities were fully aware that recreation and entertainment assisted a patient's rehabilitation and this was part of the accepted order; besides indoor and outdoor games, the superintendent's reports often mention entertainments of one type or another, sometimes procured from outside and often making use of resident talent.

Plays and concerts were arranged, originally in the dining hall and, from 1881, in the new Recreation Hall. Superintendent Gilland recorded that, on 11 August 1871, the Gower Company gave 'a musical and dramatic entertainment' to much laughter and enjoyment on the part of the patients. A later report tells that J.M. Morton's farce *Box and Cox* was performed, entirely from the asylum's own resources, on Boxing Day 1872. This, too, met with much approval. Dr Gilland, his assistant Dr Alexander Reid Urquhart, and Head Male Attendant Alfred Lockie are on record as being frequent and enthusiastic performers.

An April 1886 journal reports another successful, hired musical entertainment costing £1 11s 6d and goes on to mark the arrival of the asylum's first pianoforte. Rather than being rushed into service, and in due deference to the Powers That Be, it was placed in the luncheon room to await inspection by the Committee of Visitors during their next meeting.

December saw Wallingford Amateur Dramatic Club deliver a gratis performance to 250 persons, described as 'most enjoyable' whilst, in January 1887, at the considerable cost of 3 guineas, patients received 'a very good lecture on China and the Afghan War, illustrated with numerous magic lantern views'. Meanwhile the attendants had been provided with a dance and supper on New Year's Eve. Although this was an annual custom, Gilland had reported discontent among his employees and would have wanted to keep them 'on side'.

The festive season was a time for making special efforts to provide amusement and a good Christmas dinner. Although details have proved elusive, the BRO tells us that in 1913 there was a friends' society that assisted in decorating the hospital and providing Christmas cards and small gifts to the patients, while the staff were rewarded with roast goose.

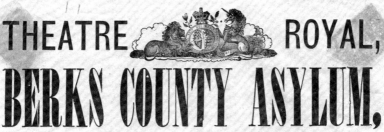

THEATRE ROYAL,

BERKS COUNTY ASYLUM,

THURSDAY, DECEMBER 26TH, 1872.

The Director and Stage Manager have pleasure in announcing the opening of the Moulsford Theatre Royal, which has been decorated in Metropolitan style by their eminent Scenic Artist, and the engagement, regardless of expense, of a brilliant staff of Amateurs, the majority of whom will appear in public for the first time this evening. The performance to-night will be under the special patronage of G. C. Cherry, Esq., Chairman of the Committee of Visitors. Notwithstanding the alarming rise in the price of coals, the charges for admission will be found consistent with the purses of the community, and the proceeds, if any, will be handed over to the Tichbourne Defence Fund.

AT 7 P.M.,

THE AREA BELLE,

An Original FARCE in One Act.

BY BROUGH AND HOLLIDAY.

CHARACTERS.

PITCHER (in the Police, with a penchant for cooks and cold mutton,) - - - - - Mr. J. C. CRUMP.
TOSSER (in the Grenadiers, a dangerous character in time of peace,) - - - Dr. R. B. GILLAND.
WALKER CHALKS (a Milkman—the devoted genuine article—no analyst required,) - - - Mr. J. G. EVANS.
Mrs. CROAKER (the " Missus," a non-political economist, with an angelic temper,) Mrs. H. M. HORTON.
PENELOPE (the " Area Belle," a charming creature, but with an extravagant taste for " lovyers,") Mrs. C. A. GOLDING.

AT 8.30 P.M.,

BOX AND COX,

A Romance of Real Life in One Act.

BY JOHN MADISON MORTON, Esq.

CHARACTERS.

JOHN BOX (a Journeyman Printer,) - - - - - Dr. R. B. GILLAND.
JAMES COX (a Journeyman Hatter,) - - - - Mr. J. C. CRUMP.
Mrs. BOUNCER (a Lodging-house Keeper,) - - - Mrs. C. A. GOLDING.

Scenic Artist—Mr. Lorhowhedanbs.   Stage Manager—Mr. J. C. Crump.

Doors open at half-past Six o'clock.

CHILDREN IN ARMS AND WET UMBRELLAS NOT ADMITTED.

Carriages to be ordered at Eleven. Horses heads to face the Moon.

Printed at W. D. JENKINS'S Machine Office, Wallingford.

Box and Cox poster. (Reproduced by permission of the Berkshire Record Office)

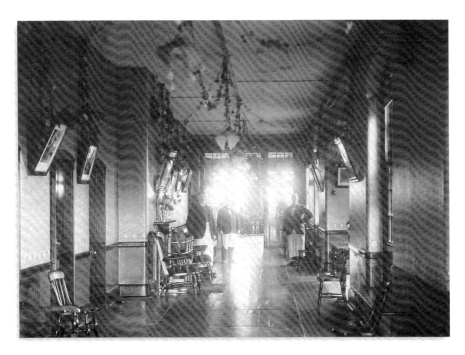

Christmas in either Male 8 or Male 9 in about 1913. Seen from the gallery, with the day room beyond. (Spackman collection)

Under Superintendent Douty, indeed from his first monthly report of March 1887, we learn that steps were taken to form a choir from among the patients and staff 'for use in the Chapel and at the Weekly Entertainments'. This is slightly mysterious, as choir practice was mentioned by the chaplain as early as 1870. Adding variety, a conjuror named Seaton 'gave a good and very amusing entertainment' on 6 April 1887 and in August, in keeping with the customs of the countryside, a Harvest Home supper was organised for patients who worked on the farm.

Over time, the stage of the Recreation Hall also hosted amateur thespians from Cholsey. An active contributor in this way was Revd Sheehan, vicar of Cholsey from 1940–45, who did a great deal of fine work with young people. 'The Vicar's Group' is still remembered for its pantomimes and we are fortunate to have a picture of a full cast, all of whom can be named.

Royal occasions were an excellent reason to splash out and, marking Queen Victoria's Golden Jubilee on 20 June 1887, the entertainments included 'athletic sports with a large number of useful and acceptable prizes for the events'. There was also a dance in the hall and 'Glees and Choruses by the staff, of appropriate nature'. A budget of £5 was allocated, the final cost being a commendable £4 5s 5d. Costs had soared by June 1911, when £15 was set aside to celebrate the coronation of King George V.

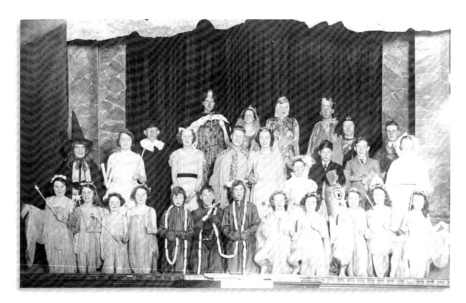

'The Vicar's Group', led by Revd Sheehan, performed plays in the village and at the BMH, as here in around 1940. This was *Sleeping Beauty*. Rear (elevated) from left: Mr Hitchins; Mrs Barnard; Mrs Beaumont; Gerald Woolley. Standing: Dick Vickery; Vi Hearmon; J.R.F. Davis; Celia Gibbs; John Money; Eileen Gibbs; Ron Brasher; Peter Basher; Alan Barnard; Ray Beasley; Roddy Hutt; Kathy Rumble. Kneeling: Edna Wyatt; Alice 'Betty' Hawkins; Edna Crook; possibly Margaret Bryant; Donald Valentine; Fred Ebsworth; Donald 'Donkey' Brewerton; Marina Heath; Daphne Howse; Jeanne Wheeler; Margie Woolley; Barbara Butler. Ron Brasher was a wartime evacuee from London, while Donald Brewerton was an upholsterer at the BMH. Vi Hearmon was very popular for her singing voice. (Spackman collection)

Although no budget was mentioned for celebrating the next coronation, that of King George VI in May 1937, the occasion coincided with the visit of Commissioners J. Coffin Duncan and H.C. Devas, who noted:

> The grounds, which are looking at their best at this time of year, are charm-ingly decorated with bunting and flags and the majority of patients are wearing loyal emblems. A special diet is to be provided tomorrow and there is a long programme of sports and other entertainments.

Peace Celebrations

The passage of a century has inevitably softened the trauma and agonies of 'the war to end all wars' but we can still imagine the nation's enthusiasm for the official Peace Day celebrations on 19 July 1919. It is known that local female revellers dressed up as servicemen, while men donned skirts and make-up before everyone paraded through the streets of Wallingford, meaning that the accompanying photo probably shows a contingent from the Berkshire Mental Hospital on that joyful day.

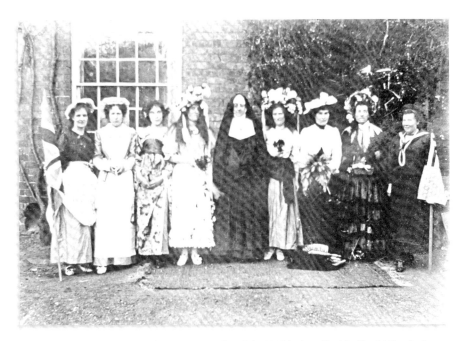

Cross-dressing for the Peace Celebrations of 19 July 1919 is described in David Beasley's *Wallingford at War* and this group from the Berkshire Lunatic Asylum was probably photographed in Wallingford. Note the Union Jack and Stars & Stripes flags. Second from left is Mary Ratcliffe, who was by this time Head Female Nurse. (Spackman collection)

Reading Matter

Books and other reading material were provided from a very early date, the role of librarian falling upon the chaplain, who distributed books to the wards when necessary. From time to time, the Commissioners were moved to suggest that stocks be renewed and expanded, as in November 1939, when Commissioner Adamson opined that 'The library is small and not very interesting to the generality of patients', but he was sensible enough to suggest that sixpenny paperback editions be purchased to supplement the hardback volumes. The subject came up again over the years, but by 1950 a library service was operated by the County Library Service and included books in braille. From 1955, there was also a library in one of the unused wards, run by the League of Friends.

Cinema

It is easy to see the attraction of entertaining patients by a means that we now take completely for granted: moving pictures. In January 1930, Commissioner Rollisham's inspection report included the timely and enlightened proposal of a cinema projector 'as this form of entertainment is so popular in similar hospitals that I venture to ask that they (the Committee of Visitors) should consider its early provision'. The next that is known of this idea comes from November 1934, when the Commissioners observed that 'A talking film apparatus is under consideration', to which they added, 'we hope that the Committee will consider the possibility of portable wireless sets in some of the wards.'

The following year, Commissioners Wilson and Devas found that the cinematograph was expected but still not in place. Lack of progress by mid-1936 was blamed on 'difficulties with regard to seating'. A projector must finally have arrived during 1939, when we hear that the Hall hosted dances, whist drives, concerts, and two cinema shows weekly. It is assumed that the unsightly projection room was tacked on to the Recreation Hall at the same time, to protect the precious and long-overdue equipment, which was operated by the hospital's electricians. In the 1950s there was a Friday afternoon showing for patients, followed in the evening by a performance for staff.

Radio

In similar vein, wireless sets arrived only after years of good intentions and cajoling. They were not yet present in all wards in July 1936 but Dr Read gave assurances that they would be supplied. Yet in May 1937, the eagle-eyed J. Coffin Duncan and H.C. Devas were only able to manage:

> We were glad to find that wards in each side of the hospital are used as club wards, where patients can sit up until 9.30 p.m. This in some measure compensates for the fact that there are a number of wards still without wireless. Patients from these wards are therefore able to enjoy listening in the Club Ward.

After the war, local electrical retailer Lionel Baldwin helped to install a 'master' radio set, connected to speakers in the wards, where a switch on the wall alternated between the Light Programme and the Home Service. He said this led to frequent squabbles.

Television

The purchase of television sets was suggested by the Commissioners in 1954 and the matter found its way into the hands of the League of Friends, which was raising funds for eight of the expensive sets in 1956. Lionel Baldwin remembers installing the necessary cables and visiting to repair the sets so frequently that he was given a master key to all the wards! The effect of TV on other forms of amusement is not hard to imagine but we know that theatre trips to Oxford were still taking place in 1960.

Dances

Until something went haywire in the 1960s, 'proper' social dancing was second nature to most and it was natural that dances were held at the asylum. This challenged the general policy of strict segregation of the sexes but, in the 1880s, there was weekly dancing on the front lawn in clement summer weather.

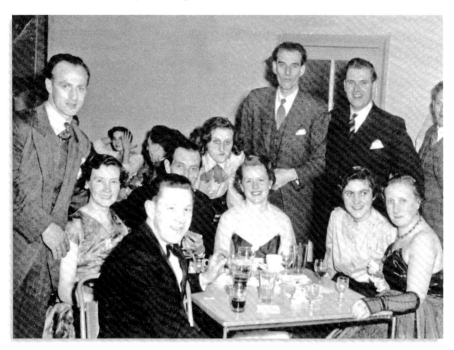

A glittering occasion for Fair Mile staff in about 1950. Tom Shorten standing left; Charge Nurses Lem White and Dick Nicholls standing tall at rear. Instructor Fran DeCondé leaning forward at centre. (Bill Nicholls)

DANCES WITH WOLVES

After the Second World War, there were dances on Monday evenings in the Villa. Vera, the attractive daughter of Hall Porter Leslie Talbot, was at that time working as secretary to Matron Hodges and was somewhat put out to be told that her duties included attending these dances, so that the visiting men had partners. As things turned out, there was nothing plural about 'partners' for Vera, since one male patient insisted on dancing with her to the exclusion of all others – and reportedly not at all well. The unfortunate man reeked of paraldehyde (a sedative and anticonvulsive) and his smile was all too easily interpreted as a leer. Vera took drastic measures to avoid such excessive attention and quit her job not long afterwards.

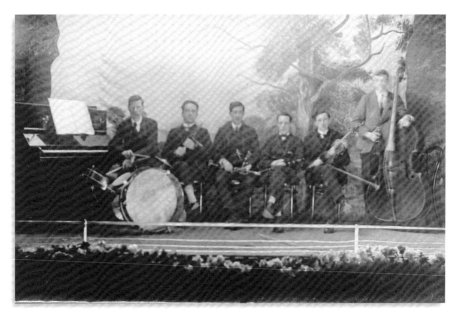

The BMH's band in around 1920. The violinist is Cyril Pryce. (The late Gwilym Pryce)

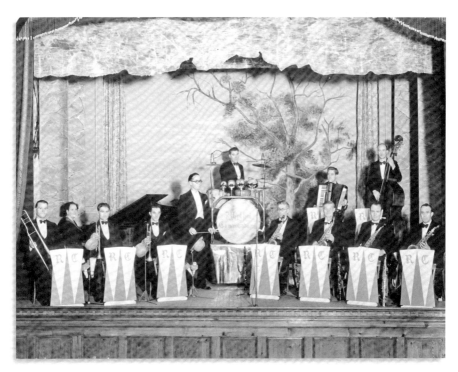

The BMH's own Rhythm Commanders on stage in about 1940. Mervyn Lovegrove, trombone, far left; Wilf Marshall on trumpet, seated third from left. The tattered 'teaser' above the players is also noticeable in the pantomime photo on page 122. (Rod Wilkins)

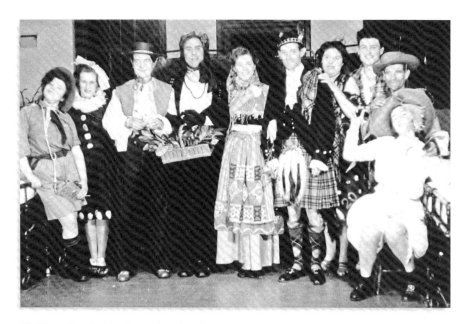

BMH staff ready for a fancy dress ball in about 1940. (Bill Nicholls)

Formal dances were held four times a year in the 1930s and, aided by advances in medication, were established twice-weekly events by the end of the 1940s. Segregation had long been relaxed for special occasions, when much care would go into dressing trusted patients in the finest clothes available, staff sometimes lending their own things. The regular New Year dance was timed to end well before midnight, so that the staff could go on to their own parties at the appointed hour. The BMH was the venue of choice for dances in the Second World War years, having the largest hall in the district, a well-maintained dance floor and its own band. These high-class events, sometimes in fancy dress, are still remembered with great affection

Miss Fair Mile

At a time when beauty pageants were seen as an amusing diversion, rather than the hyper-competitive angst-fests that had given them a bad name by the end of the twentieth century, Fair Mile held its own contest for members of staff. The only known Miss Fair Mile Dance was in May 1974. As the accompanying picture shows, Fair Mile's nursing staff were truly multi-racial by this time. Sadly, the name of the winner is not known.

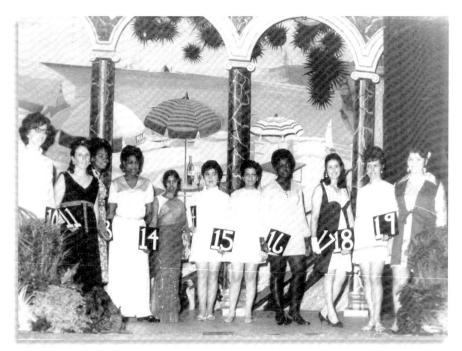

The only known Miss Fair Mile dance was on 24 May 1974. Conchita Polley is holding number 4. (Conchita Polley)

Exercise

Supervised patients took fresh air and exercise outside the wards in the airing courts. These were surrounded by a ha-ha (or ditch) and then a wall. The wall was not tall enough to spoil the view from the court but could not be scaled from the bottom of the ha-ha. Despite vigilant supervision, escape attempts sometimes succeeded, resulting in the walls being raised by Boshers, the local building firm.

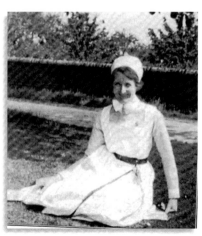

Charge Nurse Irene Wyatt in one of the Female airing courts in the 1920s. Note the ha-ha beyond the path. From the bottom of this, it was very hard to climb over the wall; meanwhile, the view of the kitchen garden was not blocked. (The late Gerald Wyatt)

Special attention had to be paid to 'noisy patients', as pointed out by Commissioner Herbert C. Bailey in May 1929, when he examined the courts. He pointed out the potential for damage or injury, 'there being a good many stones quite large enough to be used as missiles lying about'.

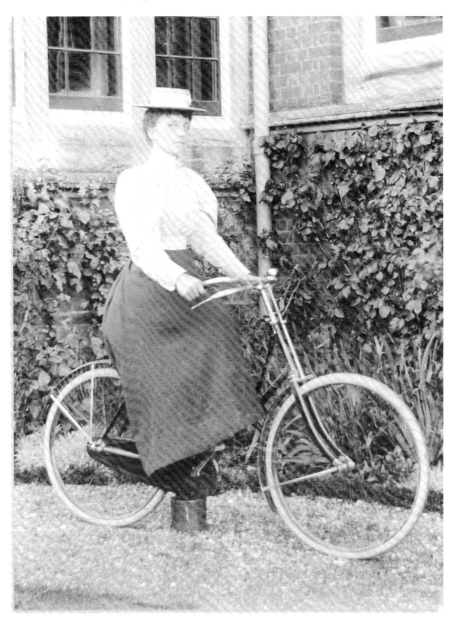

This lady taking exercise is not a patient. In fact she is believed to be Mrs Celia Murdoch, the young wife of Superintendent William Murdoch. The picture is from about 1895. (Spackman collection)

Supervised walking parties outside the hospital were established practice from at least the mid-1930s. Villagers became quite familiar with these groups and knew some patients by name. With due respect to all concerned, there was no mistaking a 'crocodile' of Fair Mile patients, who were instantly recognisable by the unfortunate effects of drugs on their expressions and gaits.

Holidays

It proved possible to give patients an occasional break from hospital surroundings. From the Commissioners, we know that in 1935 'Expeditions to the neighbouring country by motor bus have been carried out for many patients, who enjoy a picnic tea which they take with them' and it was hoped that this would extend to all patients who were fit. Seaside trips for 'working' patients were taking place by 1949 and a Fair Mile Newsletter of April 1974 also tells us that groups of patients appreciated the comfort and stimulation of a week's visit to the Royal Court Holiday Home at Clevedon in Somerset. Summer outings could be selected by the individual wards.

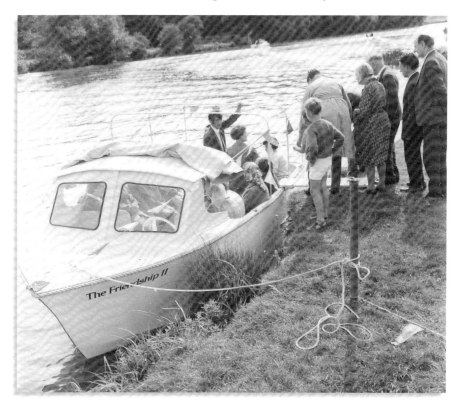

Patients taking a boat trip on the Thames, which runs past Fair Mile's grounds. The date is about 1970 and, with a name like *Friendship II*, the boat might have been provided by the League of Friends. (Spackman collection)

Garden Fêtes

The hospital's well-run garden fêtes, besides tending to be rather larger than those organised in the nearby villages, were good opportunities for patients to interact with their neighbours. Especially in the Fair Mile era, they were an annual event and sometimes organised on a lavish scale, with bands, games for adults, bouncy castles and rides for children. As late as 2002, the day's attractions included the arrival of a Puma helicopter from nearby RAF Benson and displays of vintage motor transport.

Sport

Not surprisingly, outdoor games and sports were regarded as therapeutic and were arranged from the earliest days of the Moulsford Asylum. The hospital developed a proud sporting tradition over its 133 years, not least in football and cricket.

The original cricket field existed before 1883; there were games twice weekly in the season, with informal matches on every fine evening in summer. Up to the time of the Second World War, the cricket field occupied the northern corner of the grounds, close to the farm and the Reading Road. Surrounded by Marnock's elegant parkland and with very little traffic noise from the turnpike road, this would have been a pleasant setting in which to hear the thwack of leather on willow.

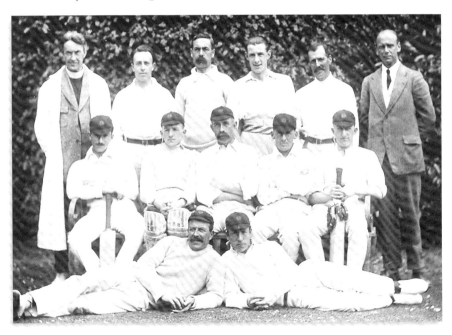

A BMH cricket team in around 1922. Back row from left: Revd Philip E. Raynor, Chaplain; Leslie Talbot, Hall Porter; Bill Southby, Clerk of Works; Bert Wooldridge; Chris Carter, Farm Bailiff and Dr Read, Medical Superintendent. Middle Row: 2nd from left, probably Archie Barnett; 2nd from right, Gerald Woolley. Front: Arthur 'Pop' Swain on the left. (John Talbot)

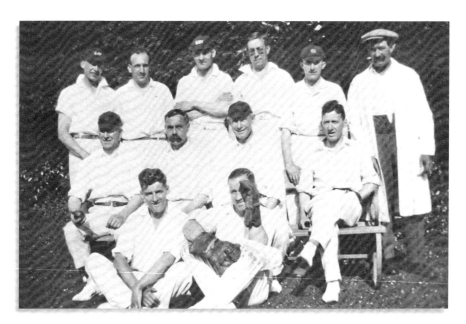

BMH cricket team in the 1930s. Back row from left: 'Strad' Challenor; unknown; unknown; J.R.F. Davis; Archie Barnett; Jack Hutt. Middle row: 'Pop' Swain; Bill Southby; unknown; Gerald Woolley. Front row: Roly Abbots; unknown. Bill Southby was Clerk of Works from 1917 to 1939. (Spackman collection)

After the war Mr Smithers, the farm manager, set out a first-class cricket field on the former kitchen gardens at the rear of the hospital. His manicured turf hosted many visiting teams, including some of the star players of the Marylebone Cricket Club, and the Fair Mile team was widely respected until it disbanded in 1995. A pavilion was erected on a corner of the field in about 1957, financed by the hospital's League of Friends, and appears to have served the needs of both cricket and football. It was rescued from a state of dilapidation during redevelopment of the site and is now in regular use by the Cholsey Cricket Club.

Football was played on a pitch by the Reading Road/Ferry Lane crossroads. The asylum's team won its first match – at home against Cholsey – in June 1872; the goalposts are visible in the aerial photograph on page 134. An adequate history of Fair Mile Hospital Football Club's exploits would demand a book of its own and the team enjoyed considerable success over many years. Patients and staff teamed up, playing at home and away against other hospitals and later expanding their horizons in various leagues, with some headline victories in the 1980s. A selection of team photographs is presented below as testament to their achievements.

In 1929, to make way for a new house for the superintendent, the pitch was relocated behind the north end of the main hospital, directly opposite the Bungalow. The whole of the original pitch was built on when the redundant hospital was converted to housing.

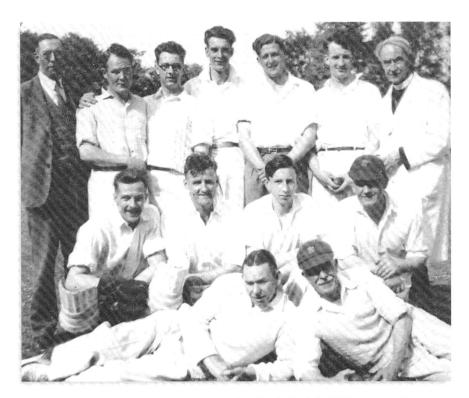

The 1947 cricket team. Back row from left: J.R.F. Davis; Earl Cecil Thompson; Lionel Carpenter; Lem White; Laurie Blake; 'Jock' Oliver; Revd Philip E. Raynor. Middle row, from left: 'Strad' Challenor; Roly Abbots; John Talbot; Gerald Woolley. Front: Fred 'Bud' Fisher, Arthur 'Pop' Swain. Philip Cecil Thompson was a very nice man, but extremely shy. He was a peer of the realm and a patient, possibly a former 'big shot' in the diplomatic service. White, Oliver, Challenor and Fisher were part of a group that came to the hospital from Creswell Colliery in Derbyshire. (Spackman collection)

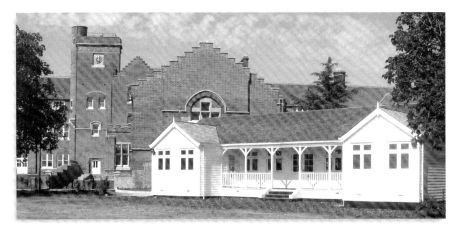

The refurbished cricket pavilion in 2014, with the Recreation Hall beyond. (Author's collection)

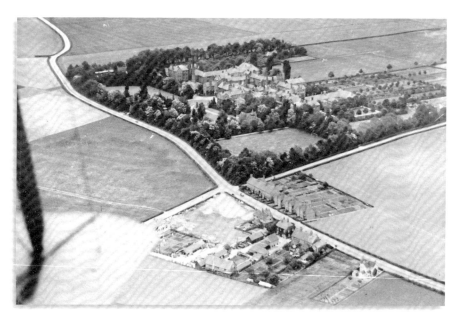

This useful view from about 1927 shows not only the football field beyond the crossroads but also the old cricket field (upper left), the kitchen gardens (upper right), Ferry Cottages and Boshers' yard on the near side of the road. (Spackman collection)

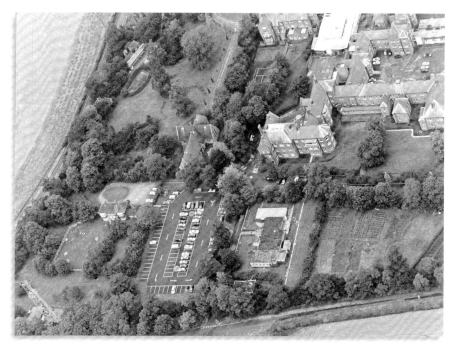

A staff car park is opposite the Fair Mile Sports and Social Club buildings in this view from around 1991. South Lodge (lower left) was being used as a crèche. Greenhouses, allotments, the tennis court and chapel can be seen. (Spackman collection)

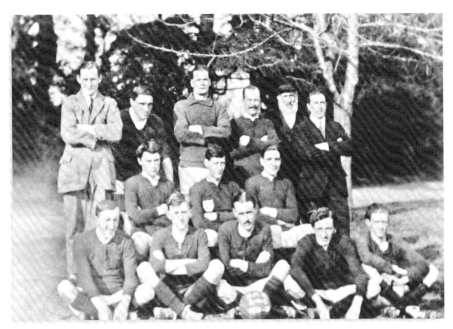

The 1922 BMH football team. Rear, 4th from left, is 'Pop' Swain. Front: 1st Archie Barnett; 2nd Jack Lambert; 4th Philip Fox. (The late Gwilym Pryce)

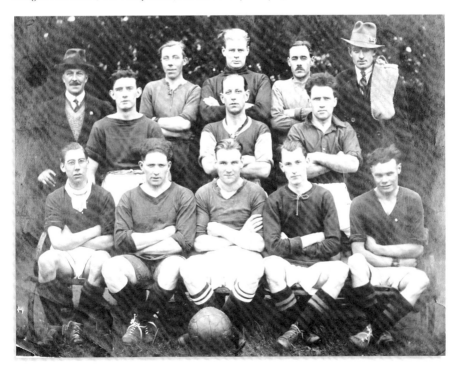

The 1942 squad. 'Pop' Swain left in hat. Perce Talbot (stoker) second left in the back row. Jack Andrews is centre in the middle row. (The late Gwilym Pryce)

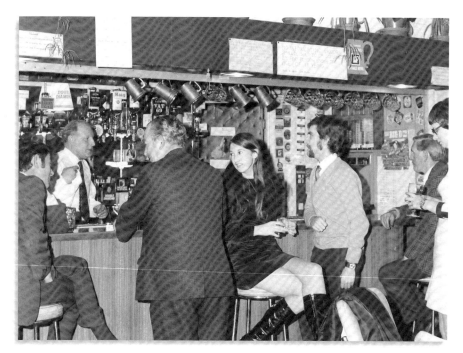

Fair Mile Hospital Social Club, around 1970. Les Collins is serving and Nick Proudlock is in a check jacket on far right stool. Anne Wood is on a stool and Rose Mundy is right. (Spackman collection)

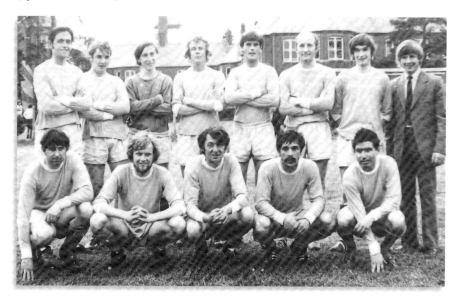

Fair Mile Hospital FC Upper Thames Inter Hospital League Winners 1971. Back row: C. MacDonald, J. Farrow, P. Hearmon, A. Spackman, R. Wright, A. Vanninetti, C. Daly, M. Farragher. Front row: R. Ballard, M. Neal, W. Salter, R. Williams, A. Diaz. (Spackman collection)

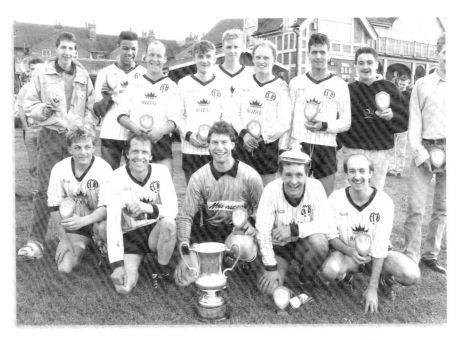

Fair Mile Hospital FC All Champions Cup Winners 1988–89. Back row: K. Taylor, J. Ferguson, R. McLaughlin, W. Glossop, M. Bonner, R. Cox, P. McDonald, N. Voller, M. Rourke. Front row: P. Everley, A. Stacey, A. Stanley, A. Taylor, M. Fox. (Spackman collection)

The Fair Mile Sports and Social Club (FMSSC) was founded in 1963, membership being compulsory for all staff members, who paid a subscription of 6*d* a week. In 1964 a generous donation from the Friends of the Fair Mile and Hungerford Hospitals enabled the opening of a large, dedicated clubhouse with bars, a function room and billiards rooms. Boshers undertook enlargement of the clubhouse in 1973. The club developed into a solid and ambitious organisation that survived the hospital's closure and, as related in Chapter 13, now owns the nearby Morning Star public house.

10

WORK AND
TRAINING

....

At the time of the asylum's creation, what we would nowadays call the nursing staff were known as 'attendants'[34]. As psychiatric care was a very new discipline, this was initially not a particularly skilled job and training was largely based on experience and the extensive Staff Regulations[35], which left few aspects of their lives uncontrolled. Paramount in these provisions was the fundamental duty of care towards patients who could not be held accountable for their words or actions, which had to be matched by a spirit of the greatest forbearance on the part of those caring for them.

It would be unfair to suggest that the job was like being a prison warder but anecdotes reveal that male attendants, who were often ex-servicemen, needed to be physically robust as violent attacks were something of an occupational hazard.

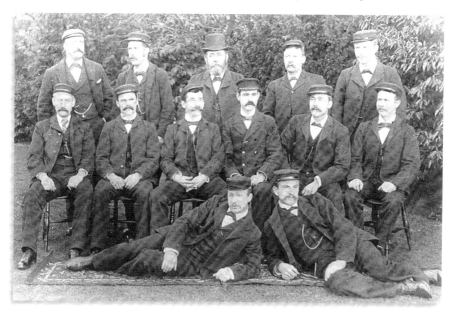

Male attendants with Head Attendant Alfred Lockie presiding. The picture may be from around 1883, when smart uniforms were first issued and moustaches appeared to be obligatory. (Spackman collection)

Stamina was also necessary since, for both sexes, the hours of work from Monday to Saturday were from 6 a.m. to 8 p.m. including a meal break, relieved to 6 a.m. to 6 p.m. on Sundays. Days off – one per month – started at 10 a.m., so the morning's chores obviously had to be done before stepping out for a little liberty.

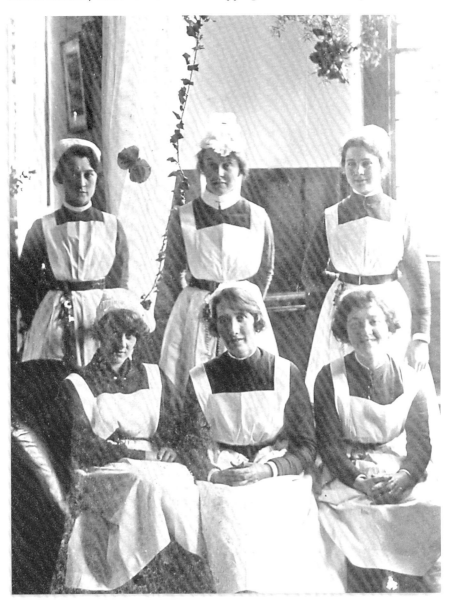

A group of BMH nurses. Rear left is Violet Newstead (later Perry); Grace Kirk is on the right. Bottom left is Rosalie Sammons, later Brignall. The hanging decorations suggest Christmas. As Grace Kirk was Deputy Charge Nurse from 1919 and her uniform here appears to be that of a nurse, this photo is likely to be pre-1919. (Spackman collection)

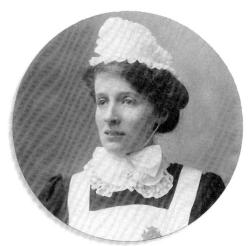

Although it is likely that this picture predates her arrival, Nurse Mary Ratcliffe came from the Salop County Asylum as Head Female Nurse in 1909. The title of 'Housekeeper' was added to this in 1927, equivalent to Matron. Her departure in 1932 was lamented by the Committee of Visitors. (Spackman collection)

In recompense, male attendants enjoyed a relatively advantageous annual salary of £20, whilst their female counterparts commanded just £17. This can be compared with £70 paid to the Head Male Attendant and the princely sum of £300 enjoyed by the Medical Superintendent. For some, notably the senior officers, there were fringe benefits – listed in staff records as 'emoluments' – in the form of accommodation, coal, lighting and produce from the asylum's farm and gardens.

The first discovered mention of training is from 1887, when Superintendent Douty proposed a series of lectures on nursing. Little more is known until the advent, in 1922, of the Registered Mental Nurse qualification (the point when 'nurse' was formally adopted[36]), which was supported by an exacting training programme that tested nurses' intelligence, discipline and resilience under pressure. Mary Fairbairn's experiences (page 145) do little more than hint at the rigours of three years' hard work.

Tough Conditions

'Living in' is mentioned earlier in this account and it was accepted practice that attendants would live on the asylum premises. Few exceptions were made until about the time of the Second World War. Staff bedrooms were situated on the wards and, considering the long working week and lack of private space, it is no wonder that there were long-term problems with recruiting and retaining good personnel.

Attendants on duty had few comforts although, in December 1886, Acting Superintendent Barron made available a mess room for use by off-duty female night staff, which was much appreciated. The same was to be considered on the Male side. Concessions of this type were well motivated but slow in appearing.

Any liberty would have been cherished but a well-intended note from Superintendent Douty on August 1887 nevertheless questioned the wisdom of allowing too much freedom:

The attention of the Committee is drawn to the evils, sanitary and otherwise, which arise from the short evening leaves (three a week) granted to Attendants in cold wet winter weather. The leave is from 8.30 p.m. to 10 p.m. every other night; and though it may be good in fine warm weather it often has bad results in winter to the health, especially of the female staff.

In July 1910 it was decided that officers and servants would not receive their board and lodging allowance (if granted) while on annual leave, which seems decidedly mean. On a more positive note, their uniform of any but the latest issue would become their property.

The following comment, made in April 1924 by the Commissioners to the Board of Control, serves to illustrate the continual problem of retaining good staff, which plagued successive superintendents and of which they often complained to the Committee of Visitors:

The nursing staff continue to work upon the basis of a 66 hour week with two days off duty weekly and an annual leave of three weeks. 40 percent of the male and 25 percent of the female nurses can show more than five years service in the institution.

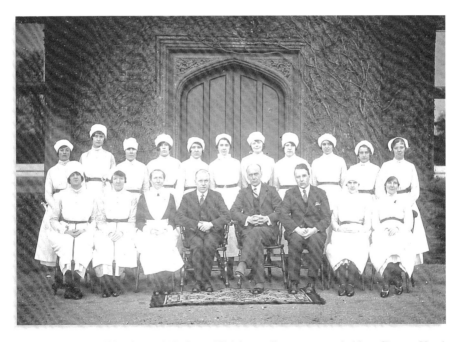

Female nursing staff in about 1930. Grace Kirk is standing centre, probably as Deputy Head Female Nurse. The severe-looking Matron is Mary Ratcliffe, who departed the BMH in February 1932. To her right is Dr Sidney Holder, First Medical Assistant; then Dr Walter Woolfe Read, Medical Superintendent. (Spackman collection)

Staffing remained a problem in 1932. There were enough men but fifty-nine female nurses left the hospital ten under strength. Some were part-time, others temporary and nurses who had left to marry were being recalled. Significantly, it fell to the Commissioners to suggest, in November 1934, that a nurses' home be provided to relieve the self-evident pressures of living in. Sadly, there was no real action on this until 1952 (see Chapter 4).

RICHARD VAUGHAN'S ARRIVAL

A respected member of the nursing staff, Richard 'Dick' Vaughan gave this account in a Fair Mile Newsletter of 1971, which he edited. Dick tells of starting at the Berkshire Mental Hospital in 1935:

I arrived in Cholsey Station at 4 p.m. About six passengers apart from myself alighted from the train and somehow disappeared before I could ask for directions to the hospital. Seeing a porter bending over a parcels truck I approached him. He looked up. 'Going up top?' he asked. The porter sensed that I hadn't understood so he changed it to 'Want the big house, mate?' After informing him that this was so, he gave me the directions and indicated that it was just over a mile. 'Any chance of a taxi?' I asked. He replied that he was afraid not – there was only Old Mont who ran a taxi and he was out. After a moment's thought he remarked 'You'll have to UFF IT'. This I gathered meant 'Hoof it – walk it' so off I trudged, lugging my case.

Through the iron gates by the porters lodge, I entered the grounds; the perfect lawns contrasting pleasantly with the gravelled surrounds and well laid out flower beds; a creeper flourished over the front of the building and curled away over the roof. All this looked so beautiful and tranquil – I found out that it was just a veneer for a drab and austere interior.

Introducing myself to the Hall Porter[37] I was soon in the presence of the Head Attendant[38] (the title of 'Nurse' came some years later). He was a kindly but gruff man who never used two words where one would suffice. He was well respected by all partly, I think, because he was always fair when dealing with staff problems and partly because he always said what he meant and meant what he said. After a short interview, I signed for a whistle, a bunch of keys and a rule book. It was emphasised that they must be handed in when I left. We then set off for my room. This entailed climbing numerous steps and finally arriving in 'Top sevens' now known as Grazeley. He opened the room door and what a depressing sight it was! The contents were:- one iron bedstead complete with rolled up flock mattress, two blankets, two sheets, two pillows and a counterpane all laid out in army fashion and covered in dust which could only have collected in weeks; one washstand with jug and basin;

one single wardrobe, the top of which was covered in masses of twigs and other nesting materials used by pigeons. There were droppings everywhere. This was the pigeons' home and I was the intruder! In addition there was a hard chair and a small carpet on an otherwise uncovered floor to complete the furnishing. The heating was non-existent.

The Head Attendant grunted something about showing me the ward and started to walk away down the stairs, tapping his key on the wall in an irritating fashion as he went. Arriving at the ward door, he opened it. I stepped inside. A voice behind me bellowed 'Another one for you, Charge!' The door slammed and he had gone, leaving me under the scrutiny of about forty patients and several staff. I felt like a specimen under a microscope.

The Charge met me, introduced himself and shook hands, then introduced the other three staff. He was a reserved type of man who, one felt, always remained composed in any situation. The three others were very friendly and helpful. One came from the North of England, one from Somerset and the other who, by the fact of being bald, was known as 'Curly' and came from London. (For some reason, no local people[39] were taken on the nursing staff in those days.)

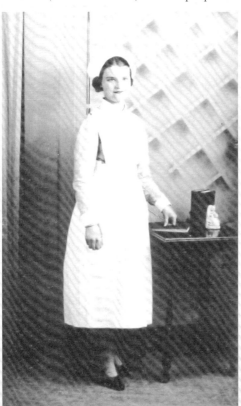

The Charge Attendant took me to one side to discuss my duties etc. (only the Head Attendant had an office). He informed me that the hours of duty were 66 hours a week including meal times which amounted to $1\frac{1}{2}$ hours per day, i.e. the first week consisted of five days from 7 a.m. to 8 p.m., and the second week consisted of four days of 7 a.m. to 8 p.m. plus one of 7 a.m. to 10 p.m., which somehow averaged 66 hours per week.

A very smartly turned-out Edith Faulkner in about 1936. She married Dick Vaughan, one of the Creswell Colliers, and was known to most as 'Blossom'. (Val Collett)

The midday meal was a cooked one, taken in the mess room, but all other meals the staff must provide themselves in the ward kitchen from 'rations' received every Wednesday afternoon. (No matter how careful one was, the so-called 'rations' never lasted more than two days and then one had to buy food.)

Except when relieved, my domain was the 'gallery'. The patients were discussed and those needing special attention for one reason or another pointed out. I was never to leave that domain for any reason without first obtaining permission from the Charge, nor was I ever to take a patient from there without permission.

It was my duty to see that each patient performed his ablutions every morning and was always tidily dressed before breakfast. The cleaning of the gallery was also one of my duties.

Whilst these instructions were being given I was wondering when he would get around to a cup of tea and something to eat. After much prompting from my stomach I plucked up enough courage to ask. The reply was shattering. There wasn't any food on the ward and he doubted whether anyone had any tea left. In any case there was nowhere to make it as all ward fires were raked out after 5 p.m. I hinted at the main kitchen but drew a blank; all the kitchen staff usually went home about 5.30 p.m. My disappointment must have registered for, as if to cheer me up, he remarked that I could always obtain bread and cheese at the pub after 8 p.m. Eight o'clock was only an hour away but it seemed ages. In the meantime, one of the staff had made my bed so, on the last stroke of eight, I hurried off to find the pub. Never did a desert traveller display more eagerness to reach an oasis than I did to reach that pub. Nor did the saliva of Pavlov's dog receive more stimulation from the sound of the bell than mine did at the thought of that bread and cheese!

Returning to the hospital at 10 p.m. (the rule book stated: 'In your room by 10 p.m. and lights out by 10.20 p.m.'), I went to bed but just couldn't get off to sleep, it was so cold. Finally, after shivering for hours and in desperation – although I knew it would be frowned upon in the best of circles – I took the solitary carpet from the floor and put it on the bed. This must have done the trick for I was sound asleep when the night roundsman hammered on my door at 6.30 a.m.

Mary Fairbairn was a contemporary of Dick Vaughan; she remembered similar working hours and that breakfast was taken on the ward at 7.00 a.m.

MARY FAIRBAIRN'S TRAINING YEARS

Before psychotropic drugs became available in the 1960s, great mental hospitals such as Fair Mile (formerly Berkshire Mental Hospital) could provide only custodial care for the mentally ill. Because unsedated patients could be combative and violent, the staff were taxed to work compassionately and professionally with them, maintaining general safety while never responding when attacked. British lunacy laws were strict regarding this, and it meant that only special people with high levels of self-control and compassion could meet the challenge of working in the field.

As a training hospital, the BMH was in the forefront of creating such people. Each new class of student nurses was endlessly evaluated to ensure they learned not only hospital practice and bedside techniques, but had the right kind of personality to work with the mentally ill. The quasi-military discipline to which these students were subject ensured that only the strongest and most suitable would survive three years to earn the title of Registered Mental Nurse.

Mary Fairbairn became one of these trainees in 1935. Her unique and entertaining account of her BMH years and her subsequent career in psychiatric nursing reveals her basic humanity, sparkling sense of humour and love of life. She tells how the students were given responsibility from the first day and held strictly accountable; this was designed to reveal any character weaknesses. Her first assignment was to watch an actively suicidal patient. Uncomfortable as yet in her brand-new uniform, Mary took off her cufflinks while she did some ward sewing. A few moments later, they had disappeared, and the patient was gleefully asking how she was going to tell Sister that the links had been swallowed. The ward sister was stern: 'Never take your eyes off a patient,' she told Mary. But she was also pragmatic. The patient got cascara, the links were retrieved and no fuss was made. Part of being a mental nurse, Mary discovered in those early days of learning ward protocols, was learning how to respond to the totally unexpected.

More serious instruction and correction came from the assistant matron. She was known to the students as The Wasp because she tried to catch them out in even the most minor of infractions – such things as incorrect preparation of an enema tray. She had perfected the art of making student nurses feel inadequate. The more serious offences meant dismissal and, more importantly, she had that power. Lesser ones, such as answering back to senior staff – possibly from the fatigue of long days of scrubbing floors, changing bedding, dressing and feeding the patients and working overtime because of staff shortages – saw the offender sent to climb a ladder to scrape pigeon droppings off the hospital cistern. Mary says she went up there at least six times, usually with a patient subject to fits of shaking to hold the ladder.

She says she could do very little scraping, so she hung on, reading love letters from a boyfriend she had hardly any time to see.

Not far into their training, the hospital's psychiatrists began lectures on the current state of the profession; students had to attend in addition to their full duty days on the wards. The lectures covered the latest theories of mental illness but always with the caution that nothing could be done for the patients beyond giving them meticulous medical and professional treatment. Mary's memories of these lectures are acute. She describes a room full of men and women still in their uniforms, busily taking notes and trying to stay awake.

With seniority came more responsibility. Back on the ward, when she was left in charge overnight, her 'ladies' knew this was her first night in charge and were not co-operative. Since nursing students slept in rooms adjoining the ward, Mary knew she could call for help but she wanted to deal with it herself. After one chaotic night, she installs a therapy of tea and broken biscuits. 'Anyone willing to keep the ward quiet tonight and help in the morning, come out for a cup of tea and a biscuit,' she calls out. It works. After that, the ward is with her and she has no more trouble. These are the tricks that only experience can teach her.

Her first day charge is just as dramatic. The patient who swallowed the cufflinks drinks Bluebell metal polish. Mary blows her emergency whistle and handles the situation as she has been trained to. When it is over, she talks severely to the student nurse assigned to watch the woman, repeating the same words the ward sister had used to her.

Mary never saw a patient mistreated at the hospital. In fact, she describes only professionalism and dedication. If cures were not available, the staff substituted meticulous care and unfailing tolerance. Popular fiction may suggest otherwise, she says, but anyone who abused patients was immediately sacked – and she saw it happen.

In fact, the nursing staff did everything they could to make the patients' lives as happy as possible. She describes how the cheery Occupation Therapy girls collected ladies from the ward for daily work or crafts. In the summer, she took small groups out into the airing yard so that they could enjoy the lovely countryside and, a couple of times a year, escorted them down to the auditorium for a dance. With everyone dressed in their best, the administrative staff made a grand entrance and patients and staff danced with one another. It was all very innocent and great fun.

Mary describes in detail the probing and thorough examinations she had to pass for her certification. These were given at national hospitals, mostly in London. Out of a class of thirty students, twelve became qualified graduate nurses.

Mary's RMN from the BMH was the basis of a career lasting fifty years. She transferred to Warren Road Hospital in Guildford, working on a psychiatric observation ward during the Blitz. From there she accepted a position at

Borocourt Mental Hospital, working with Down's syndrome men and boys. By then she had her daughter to consider, so she worked for a private nursing co-operative in Brighton, nursing famous, rich, and aristocratic patients until she was part of the wave of British medical staff that emigrated to Canada during the 1950s. There, she participated in the new treatments made possible by psychotropic drugs and the impetus to move patients out of the great mental hospitals and into their communities, a movement that is still ongoing. (Kindly contributed by Mary Fairbairn's daughter, Diana M. DeLuca, PhD.)

***

The author recommends the full and highly informative version of Mary's experiences at Fair Mile, published in 2013 by the Berkshire Medical Heritage Centre in Reading, under the title *Nursing at the Fairmile Mental Hospital, Cholsey*. Her complete memoir, which is essentially a history of modern mental nursing from the viewpoint of the psychiatric staff, is forthcoming under the title *Affairs of the Mind: My Life as a Mental Nurse*, published by Seafield House.

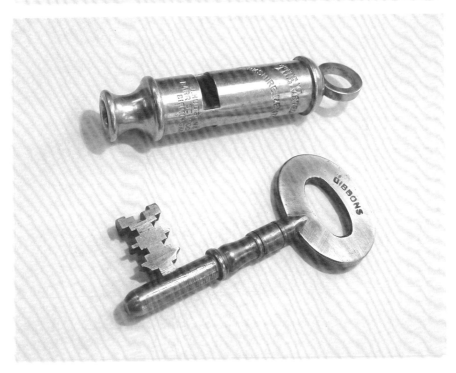

Lilian Talbot's pass key and alarm whistle. (Author's collection)

Vera Wheeler adds some further colour to the hospital's working day:

My mother, Lilian Talbot, worked there from the age of 17 (1920) until she married my father, Leslie, who was initially an attendant but subsequently became Hall Porter. Married couples were not allowed to work at the same hospital at that time. All doors were opened with keys, which had to be handed into Father's office as staff went off duty and left the building. They were collected when they reported for duty. The male attendants carried their keys in their pocket, attached to their trousers by a chain. To the best of my recollection the female nurses had theirs buttoned to their uniform on a fabric strip.

Male staff wore navy blue suits and peaked caps, much as the old prison officers wore. Female nursing staff wore a grey/blue dress, a white bib and apron and a nurse's hat. I remember seeing a picture of my mother wearing her uniform at the time she became a charge nurse – the modern term would be 'sister' – and she was immensely proud of her 'strings'; these were the ties that came from each side of the cap and tied under the chin in a bow.

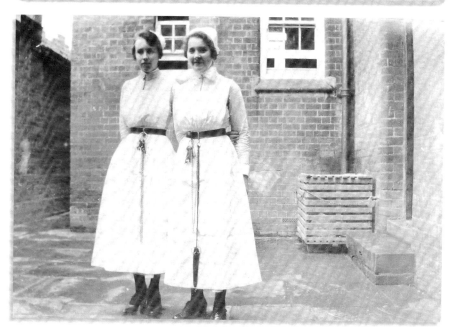

Sisters Annie and Grace Kirk in July 1925. Grace shows off her 'strings', the bow beneath the chin denoting Charge Nurse status. She was promoted to Deputy Head Female Nurse in 1926 and went on to succeed Mary Ratcliffe as Head Female Nurse and Housekeeper (Matron) in 1932. Annie married Gerald Woolley, who ran the stores, while Grace married a doctor in 1938 but sadly died young. (Author's collection)

Post-war Training

At the end of the Second World War there was a severe shortage of nurses, and interested candidates were employed from many countries, 'female staff of continental origin' being first mentioned in 1954. Even so, many of these required training in the specialised skills that had developed in psychiatric medicine. Although Fair Mile had long been a training hospital, it lacked facilities; there was a classroom in the basement of the original superintendent's quarters from 1932 but the Recreation Hall or even the operating theatre sometimes had to be pressed into service.

Moulsford Manor

The answer was the creation of a residential training school just a mile towards Reading at Moulsford Manor, an elegant country house with large, panelled rooms and pleasant gardens stretching down to the Thames. The manor already had a history and was used by Winston Churchill – presumably before it was taken over by the United States Army Air Force in 1943 – as a quiet retreat from the stresses of holding the country together and beating the Axis forces.

The Moulsford Manor School of Nursing came into being in 1956 and its students came from mental hospitals far and wide and from many nations. At various times, there were intakes from Ireland, France, Spain, Germany, Holland, Italy, Portugal, the West Indies, Scandinavia and even Latvia.

Official pictures show comfortable surroundings and good facilities. Less formal views indicate that hard study was the order of the day.

The school closed in 1994, at which time the building passed into the ownership of the famous Maxwell family.

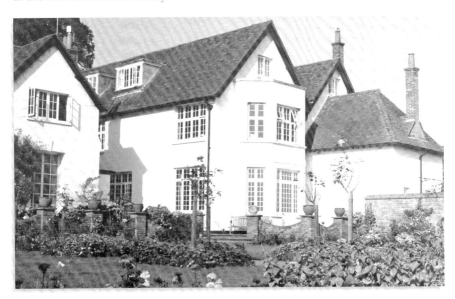

Previous page: Moulsford
Manor in the 1970s.
(Spackman collection)

Right: Momena Wright's
badge from the Moulsford
Manor training school.
(Author's collection,
courtesy of Momena
Wright)

Below: A lesson taken
in the comfortable
surroundings of
Moulsford Manor in the
1960s. Martin Morris
on the left, then Colette
Reynolds and Bill Fox.
Colette Dusaillent is
in the other corner.
(Spackman collection)

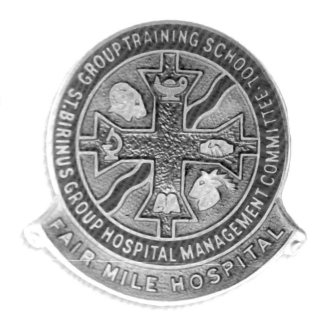

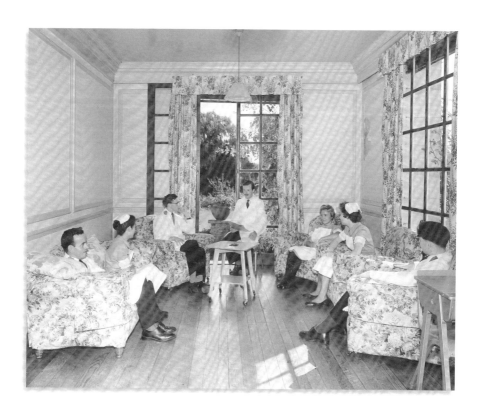

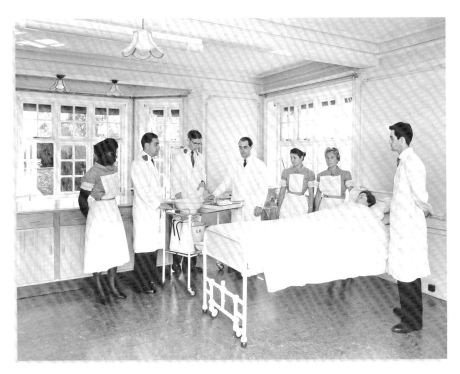

A practical session posed for the camera in the 1960s. This room was Churchill's bedroom during the war. Trainee male nurses had green lapel flashes while female trainees would not have had a badge on the bib of their apron. Bill Fox is behind the basin. Colette Reynolds and Colette Dusaillent are to the right, with Conar MacDonald far right. (Spackman collection)

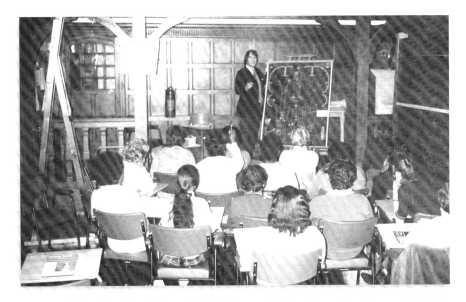

Chalk and talk at Moulsford Manor in 1972. The tutor is Alan Stirton. (Spackman collection)

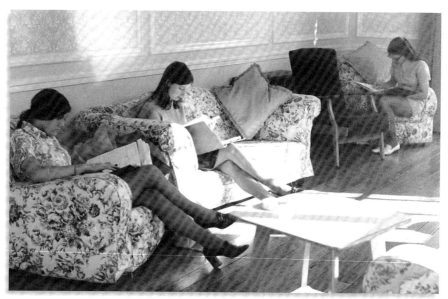

This modern-looking scene is actually from 1972. Today's students would be poring over tablet computers and smartphones. Christine Brown features on the left. (Spackman collection)

THE NIGHT RUNNER

Michael Reynolds grew up in Ferry Cottages, in Reading Road. His father, Alf, was a charge nurse and in 1956 Mike followed him into Fair Mile as a student nurse. Because he already lived in staff accommodation, he was not required to live within the hospital like other trainees.

With some amusement, Mike recalled the duties of the junior member of staff on a night shift: essentially these were any lousy tasks that were going and the unofficial job title was 'night runner' (we would probably say 'gopher' today). At the start of the shift, he had to collect heavily bound report books from the office and deliver one to each of the wards. He described staggering along the winding corridors, laden down with books in an attempt to avoid making several trips. At the end of the night, the made-up and signed books had to be returned for safe keeping.

This pales into insignificance when compared with delivering the tea, which was brewed in quantity in the kitchen at night, rather than in the ward kitchens. The poor night runner was required to deliver tea to all the staff, in all parts of the hospital, in strict order of seniority. No record exists of the miles involved in first serving all the senior personnel before repeating the tour to serve their immediate subordinates, and so forth. Suffice to say that the night runner's tea was seldom warm when he or she got it.

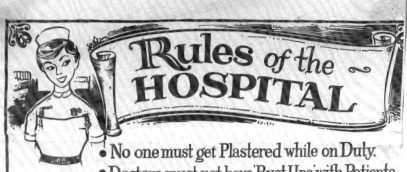

Rules of the HOSPITAL

- No one must get Plastered while on Duty.
- Doctors must not have 'Bust Ups' with Patients.
- No Short 'Cuts' to be taken to the Theatre of Operations.
- Troublesome Patients will be Bound, Gagged, Bandaged... and sold as Egyptian Mummies.
- Night Nurses must not burn the Candle at Both Ends ~ ... cut it in Half.
- Never chase after a Racing Pulse ~You can't Beat it !
- If anyone Complains about the Food-Drip feed them.
- Buckets of Cold Water must not be thrown over Patients with High Temperatures.
- If you can't lift your Patient ~ be Patient.
- Crutches must not be Worn in Bed.
- If it Moves... *Chart It !*
- Save Water...Put Two in a Bath.
- Nurses when busy, must refrain from walking on the Ceiling.
- Parties must not be held under the Blankets.
- Connecting Doors between Male and Female Wards... must be Locked at All times.
- Artificial Limbs must be hung on the Bedpost overnight. *(but not on Xmas Eve)*
- Any Nurses Roller-Skating through the Wards at Night ...*will be dismissed at Dawn*.

MOTORISED WHEEL CHAIRS must keep to the LEFT except when Overtaking

STRETCHER CASES must NOT be left in the LUGGAGE ROOM

DO NOT use LAUNDRY SHUTE for EMERGENCY CASES

A lighter look at the staff regulations, found during 2010. (Bill Nicholls)

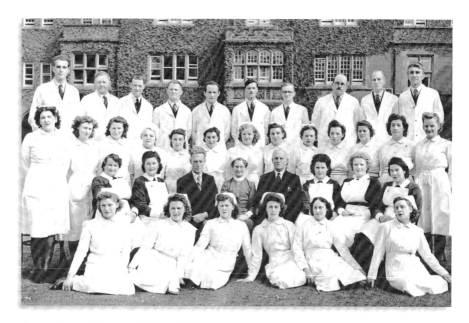

An excellent staff group of about 1951:

Rear, from left: 1st Lem White; 3rd Bert Lines; 4th Mervyn Lovegrove; 6th Bill 'Taff' Walker; 7th Bill Mundy; 8th Basil Mann. Far right: Arthur 'Lofty' Bryant.

Standing: 1st Kay Hazlewood; 2nd Ruth Green; 4th Mrs. Franks; 10th Carmel Parkinson (née Clancy); 11th Peggy Veloso (née Norris); 12th May Lehaney (later Walsh).

Seated: 3rd Arthur Perry; 4th Agnes Pilgrim; 5th John William 'Jack' Croxford (Head Male Attendant); 6th Mary Nicholls; 9th May O'Reilly.

Front row: 3rd ? Max-Deans; 5th Rees Hughs. Far right Irene 'Renee' Gorman (later Brewerton). (Bill Nicholls)

11

TRAGEDY, DEATH AND SPIRITUAL CARE

. . . .

The Chaplains

In his tenure from 1870 to 1872, **Revd George W. Oliver** worked a pattern of 11 a.m. and 6 p.m. services in the chapel on Sundays, morning prayers in the dining hall on most weekdays, followed by visiting the sick and touring the wards to talk with a high proportion of the patients. Choir practice is first itemised on Saturday, 9 December 1870.

Revd D.B. Binney was the incumbent from September 1872 to June 1875, followed by **Revd C.F. Thorndike** until 1876. **Revd W. Kirkby** was another short-term holder of the chaplaincy until November 1878, when **Revd A.O. Taylor** filled in until April 1879. The hospital was subsequently sorry to lose the services of **Revd Richard William Perry Circuitt AKC** (Associate of King's College) in 1886, after seventeen years of commendable service. He was also vicar of Cholsey.

Next was a short period in which **Revd A.L. Crake** was assisted by **Revd F.W. Agassiz**, who was curate at Cholsey and who was himself briefly Chaplain from June 1887 to October 1888. Regrettably, Agassiz was a serial philanderer and gambler, who absconded to South America.[10] **Revd Hayman Cummings** covered most of 1889 but August of that year to the start of 1896 enjoyed continuity under **Revd Augustus Edward Farrar**.

From 1896, when **Revd F.T. Stewart-Dyer** took the chaplaincy, a typical day's entry would read, 'Visited the wards, except Female 1 and 6 bathing, Laundry, Airing Courts & Workshops and conversed with many of the patients individually,' this last being perhaps linked to the customary duty of distributing library books. Failing health prompted Revd Stewart-Dyer's resignation.

In July and August 1909, we know only that **Curate H. Daman** acted as locum tenens to Stewart-Dyer during his holiday but we take a little more detail from the hand of 30-year-old **Revd G.L. Edwardes**, who arrived from the Bucks County Asylum on 30 September 1910. Although the business of his average day was little altered from that of his predecessors, he was expected to take an active part in the

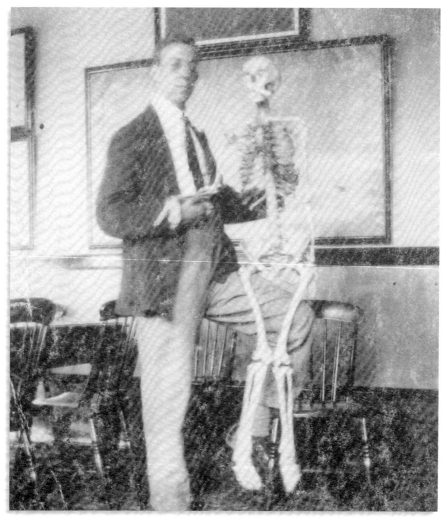

Rather than a picture of Revd Raynor, who appears elsewhere, this is the steady-looking J.R.F. Davis, long-serving finance officer and amateur thespian. Perhaps he had been taking lessons in ventriloquism from the chaplain! (Miriam Pryce)

social life of the asylum and appears to have done so with considerable energy, frequently singing solo in the weekly entertainments and leading the choir. On Sunday, 13 November 1910, there was a 'Vocal & Organ Recital' attended by 130 patients, ten attendants and three servants. The organ was played by Mr. A.G. Letts and included items by Guilmant, Lyle and Freyer. Vocal contributions were made by Edwardes himself and Miss Hilda Deacon. Edwardes was subsequently sick-listed for four days. Undaunted, he also 'attended minstrel practice', took solos in many other events and dutifully presented himself at at least one staff ball, in February 1911. He later took the peaceful-sounding curacy of Ottery St Mary in Devon.

Revd Philip Edwin Raynor AKC, also vicar of Moulsford, held the post of Chaplain from 1912 until the journals cease in 1953, shortly after the loss of his wife and when he was himself not very well. Before taking holy orders, he had been on the stage as a ventriloquist and still gave 'Tommy', his dummy, the occasional outing. He was an accomplished academic and sportsman, featuring in some of the finest older photographs, typically of cricket teams. He became friendly with authoress Agatha Christie and would play chess with her at her home in nearby Winterbrook.

All of these gentlemen were engaged at a salary of £200 per annum, typically with lunch and beer on Sundays.

There is a gap in the records after 1953 although it is known that **Revd John Hall** had the post from 1983–92, succeeded by **Revd Andrew Petit**, the last chaplain and still vicar of St Mary's, Cholsey, at the time of writing.

Although the chaplains were very much involved in the wellbeing of patients, their journals are incomplete and contribute little of historical interest, being suitable for inspection by the Committee of Visitors on a monthly basis and signed off as satisfactory. Morning prayers may have been discontinued when the sheer number of patients necessitated taking breakfast in the wards. Time was found for at least one service in the chapel on Sundays and the chaplain always recorded the numbers of those who attended. Sadly, the journals are dry and repetitive, with little opportunity to gauge the personalities of the writers. Even records of the many funerals at which the chaplains officiated are perfunctory, the tragedy being that there were often very few mourners present.

At various times, services were rescheduled to be more convenient for one or other of the hospital's functions, although the underlying aim was to maximise attendance; the chapel was twice enlarged as patient numbers grew, and suffered its own tribulations over such matters as heating. Now redundant, the building stands firm under a preservation order but its construction makes future use an interesting challenge.

Other Faiths

Naturally enough, the resident chaplain was Church of England but arrangements were also made for other denominations. No arrangements would have been necessary for any of the non-European faiths until well into the NHS era.

Death and its Causes

Death was a matter of constant concern to the staff, who were charged with preserving life where this was humanly possible. In the earlier years, many deaths were a sad result of the depleted condition of patients on arrival. Senile decay, erysipelas, general paralysis, senile gangrene, 'brain disease' (often meaning tumours), circulatory problems and pneumonia figured large, while others succumbed to diseases contracted within the establishment and there were periods when tuberculosis, enteric fever, dysentery and even the dreaded typhoid fever claimed the lives of more patients – and occasionally staff – than any self-respecting doctor could pass as routine.

For the year 1933, the causes of 164 deaths were heart disease, forty-two; senile decay, forty-two; bronchitis, sixteen; epilepsy, nine; pneumonia, five; malignant disease, five; tuberculosis, three; and general paralysis only two, the remaining forty being due mainly to natural causes. There were six cases of TB but the Commissioners felt that the hospital was 'singularly free from this disease'.

The death rate was regularly above the national average for asylums but was often explainable by the large numbers of elderly patients, including transferees from outside the area. Mortality statistics were scrutinised, particularly where a post-mortem examination was warranted, and successive superintendents clearly felt a sense of personal responsibility, reflected in the distressed tone of some of their journal entries.

By December 1938, the main causes of a 10 per cent mortality rate were organic brain diseases and cardiovascular or respiratory disorders. The national average of 7.5 per cent was achieved in 1940.

Suicides

The first suicide noted in the journals was a male patient who drowned himself in April 1872. The next was in November of the same year: it was a woman who had been discharged days earlier as unlikely to make further improvement. The risk of suicide was present throughout the asylum's history, although excellent training and vigilance on the part of nursing staff made it an uncommon occurrence. The Staff Regulations of 1904 contained clear and strict directives for the supervision of suicidal patients, foremost among these being that actively suicidal patients should never be out of the sight of nursing staff. In the 1930s, such cases were 'red carded' while patients who had not attempted self-harm in six months were 'yellow carded' and those who had only expressed intent got a green card. All were kept away from any possible means of self-harm.

Suicides nevertheless occurred and anyone who knew Fair Mile Hospital up to its latest days could be forgiven for associating the grim subject with the River Thames, which flowed along the asylum's border, and with locally named 'Silly Bridge', a lofty bridge that crosses the London–Bristol main line barely half a mile from the asylum's gates. Needless to say, the means of achieving the unthinkable were many and diverse but invariably tragic. Records of such events are largely closed to public scrutiny but readers may care to refer to *Crime and Calamity in Cholsey*, by Barrie Charles, which describes in detail a few of the earliest suicides.

Enlargement of Cholsey Churchyard

There was a disagreement – indeed, a heated dispute – in about 1908 between Revd Henry C.B. Field, the vicar of St Mary's, Cholsey, and the Committee of Visitors at the Berkshire Lunatic Asylum over the cost of burying its patients. The problems were real enough, since the asylum's death rate was more than double that of the village and the available space in the churchyard was fast dwindling. In the face of vigorous opposition from the Visitors to the spending of public money, it fell to Mr Morland, long-serving Clerk to the Visitors, to point out that the asylum had previously supported an enlargement of the graveyard in response to need and that a precedent had thus been established. There ensued a protracted and complex argument over proposals to create a new graveyard at the asylum, counter-proposals to expand the church's burial ground and quibbling over every detail of the execution of that plan. In the event, a considerable extension was created at St Mary's, which served asylum and parish alike, the costs being shared.

This wrangle being at last settled, one can only guess at the mood of the Visitors when, in August 1909, they received a letter from an unabashed Revd Field, who was 'desired' by the Committee for the Repair & Restoration of the Church Tower, to ask for a contribution from the asylum. As the asylum had willingly paid – among other amounts – half of the recent consecration expenses, they replied that they felt they had no power to make a contribution towards the tower. Whatever the final outcome on this particular affair, a journal entry of 1912 tells that the tenders for erection of a wall for the extended churchyard were submitted to the Visitors for approval and that the job fell to the respected local firm of Boshers, for the princely sum of £105.

Grave Markers

The graveyard plots in the allotted part of the churchyard had to be reused after a decent interval and very few patients' graves were graced by a headstone. Instead, iron stakes topped with a simple iron cross and a number were all that stood to remind the world of the souls who had died in the hospital. This may, in part, illustrate the inability of surviving relatives to come to terms with mental illness in the family. In some cases, of course, there were no relatives and an asylum burial was a bleak and sorry entry in the chaplain's journal. The only consolation was that most of the deceased had reached a ripe old age.

Over time, even the simple markers were progressively removed – no doubt being a serious obstacle to the mowing of the churchyard. A few still exist, stored in the parish council's shed.

There remains a beacon of remembrance and respect towards those unfortunate enough to have passed away in the asylum. At his explicit instruction, Dr James William Aitken Murdoch, much-respected Medical Superintendent from 1892 to

1917, was interred in the area set aside for asylum burials, watching over many of his erstwhile charges. Mary Fairbairn was quick to notice this when she arrived as a trainee nurse in 1935 and used the lesson in developing the skills and disciplines of her craft. Many years later, in 1962, Murdoch's widow, Celia, joined the good doctor.

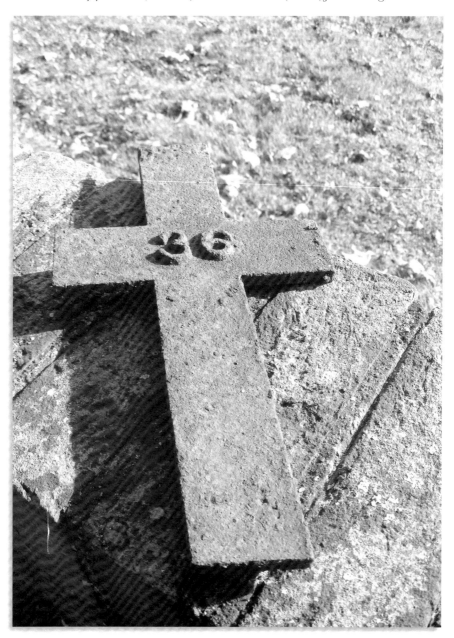

Part of a grave marker from the asylum's section of Cholsey churchyard. (Author's collection)

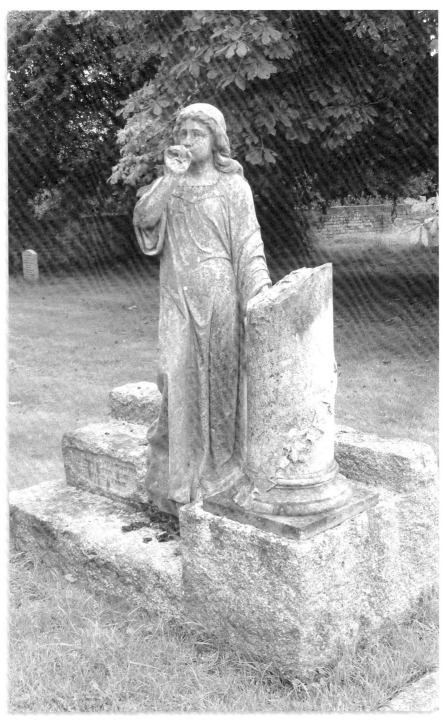

The grave of Dr James William Aitken Murdoch and his wife, Celia, watches over many
asylum patients in Cholsey churchyard. (Author's collection)

12

FADING
INTO MEMORY

∙∙

It may be rather obvious that this account has not related much detail of the NHS era – the period that introduced the name Fair Mile – but the remainder of this book's title, *A Victorian Asylum*, is perhaps what most interests the modern eye. Between 1870 and 1948, psychiatry became a well-developed discipline, society and healthcare underwent cataclysmic changes and therapeutic drugs began to alter the very nature of treatment, presenting a post-war image that was much closer to today's pill-popping[41] approach to therapy. The greater resources of the NHS permitted attempts at modernisation denied by years of war and national economic restraint; the technologies employed were mature and largely reliable and these aspects are, frankly, less fascinating.

A significant problem for researchers is that, the nearer we come to the present day, the more records are restricted. Put simply, there is not a lot of material available to draw on. Also, this book is not about modern psychiatric care – which is the real story of Fair Mile's later years and a subject too vast and specialised for these pages.

We know that the hospital adopted modern methods, some of which were as much about prevention as treatment; patients were given greater liberty and more up-to-date living conditions, although the buildings themselves prevented radical improvements. Former staff invariably describe Fair Mile as a happy place to work, whatever the physical shortcomings bequeathed by its builders.

Around 1990, the hospital was clearly approaching its 'sell-by date', a victim of progress and spiralling costs. Modern therapies, including drugs, had reduced the nation's mental hospital population from around 150,000 in the 1950s to just 25,000 and Fair Mile cared for just a few hundred in premises that once housed over 1,000. Another consideration was the 1974 change in the county boundary between Oxfordshire and Berkshire. Even though it still served Berkshire, which was now considerably smaller, Fair Mile found itself, overnight, a mile or two inside Oxfordshire.

A planning document prepared by South Oxford District Council quoted just 200 inpatients by 2002 and, given these small numbers, the fabric and sheer scale of the hospital were very real sources of difficulty. Some areas had seen neither use nor adequate maintenance for years; infrastructure was outdated and inefficient;

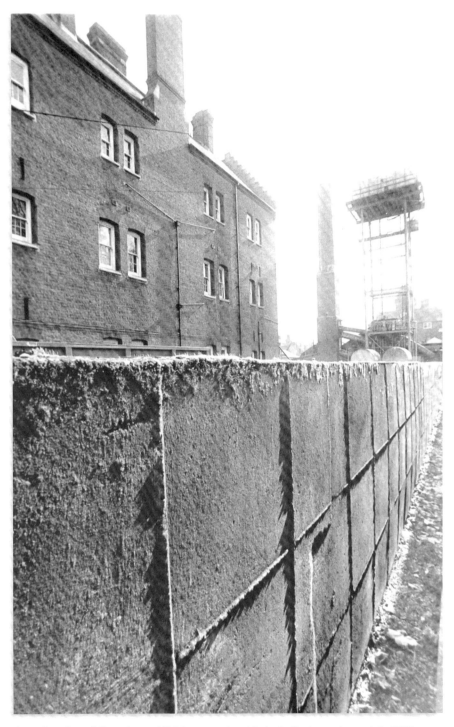

A sombre view of Grazeley and Frilsham wards, with the boiler house beyond, in 1990.
(Spackman collection)

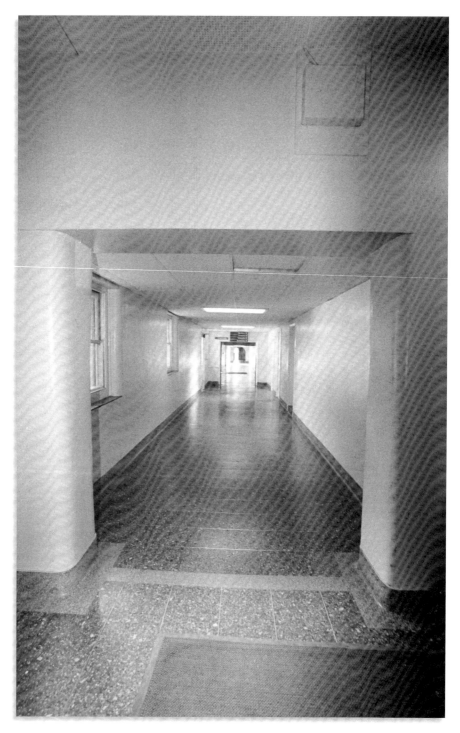

A main corridor on the Female side in about 2000. (Spackman collection)

heating the great Victorian edifice with its high ceilings and draughty corridors was costing a fortune and, despite efforts over several previous decades, the place did not lend itself to that other modern buzzword, 'upgrading'.

Tastes change, too. What had once been regarded as a handsome and rather grand establishment – comfortable surroundings if your sorrows had originated in a filthy slum or run-down cottage – was beginning to look rather stark; Marnock's mature, landscaped grounds did much to soften Howell's characteristic asylum architecture. Despite facelifts, the interiors retained their labyrinthine, tiled passageways and staircases, dormitory accommodation and chilly washrooms, which were now a far cry from the comforts of normal, modern housing.

Operating costs had become prohibitive by the 1990s, a situation possibly exacerbated by the National Health Service and Community Care Act of 1990, primarily concerned with the hocus-pocus of creating an 'internal market' for health and social care, and which resulted in a doctrine known as 'Care in the Community'. This aimed to return as many patients as possible to their home environments or, failing that, into small care units serving as a halfway house between institutional treatment and complete independence. In this development, the wheel of mental healthcare had in some ways turned full circle.

Property and land values being what they were by the 1990s, the attraction of selling off the considerable acreage of Fair Mile, even to fund a brand-new facility elsewhere, was irresistible. Although probably not the literal truth, the author was once told that a complete new hospital would cost less than one year's upkeep of the old one.

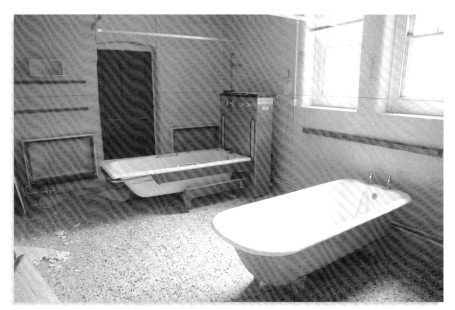

A shared bathroom. (Bill Nicholls)

In the last few years of Fair Mile's life, careful preparations were made to abandon the old homestead. Moulsford Manor had already closed and it was from there that many of the archive photographs in these pages were rescued, their significance finally appreciated. As many patients as possible were reintroduced to some semblance of a normal life in the community, while some were transferred to a purpose-built facility at Prospect Park, Reading, where the good work would continue.

The Victorian asylum closed its doors on 132 years and 7 months of service on 30 April 2003.

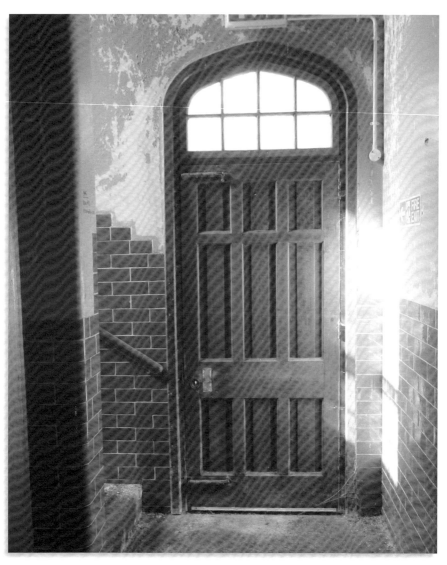

Once serviceable and fashionable, the glazed tiles in staircases and corridors took on a bleak aspect as standards of comfort changed. (Bill Nicholls)

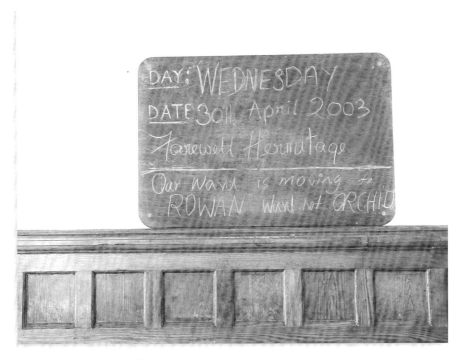

A farewell message left in Hermitage ward. (Bill Nicholls)

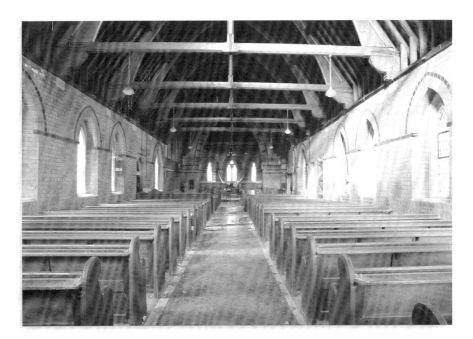

The interior of the chapel, sadly not in all its former glory in 2010. (Bill Nicholls)

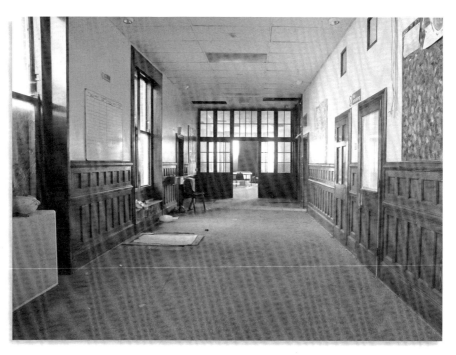

The gallery of Ipsden ward retained much of its Victorian character up to closure. (Bill Nicholls)

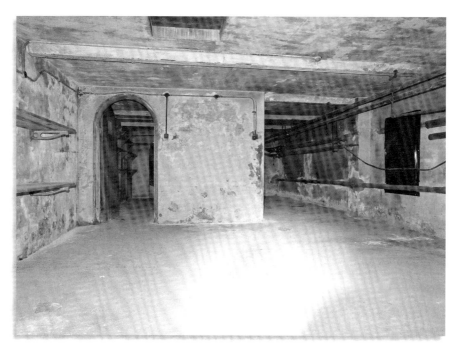

Most of the underground tunnels and chambers were filled in but this cellar survives near the site of the original kitchen. (Bill Nicholls)

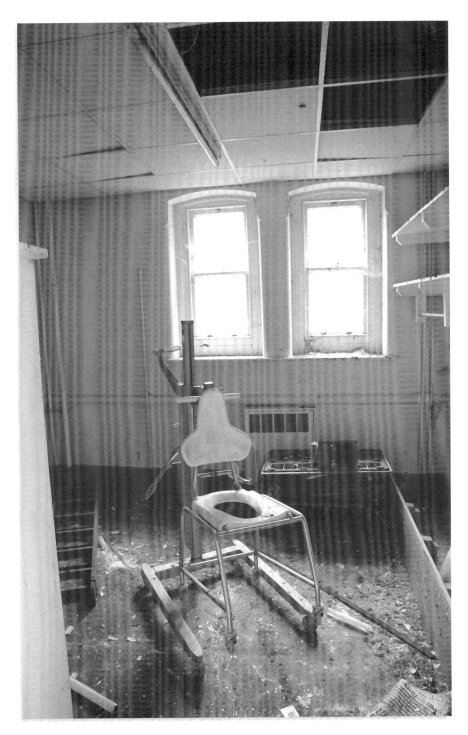

Dereliction is fascinating, although this contrivance adds a completely misleading hint of the torture chamber. (Bill Nicholls)

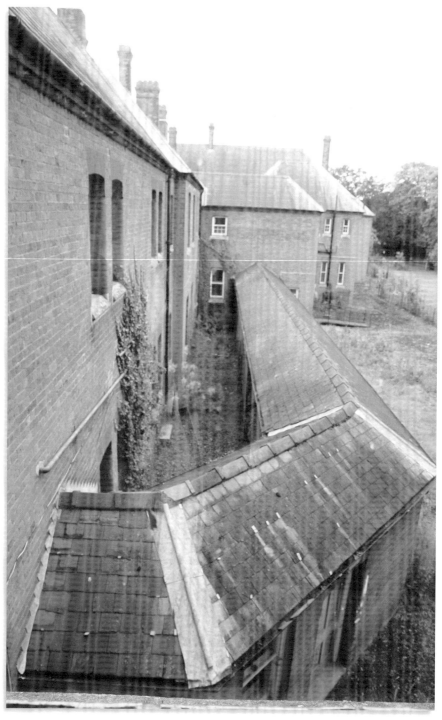

An excellent view of the external corridor serving Female 8 (Ipsden) ward. These corridors allowed discreet movement about the asylum. (Bill Nicholls)

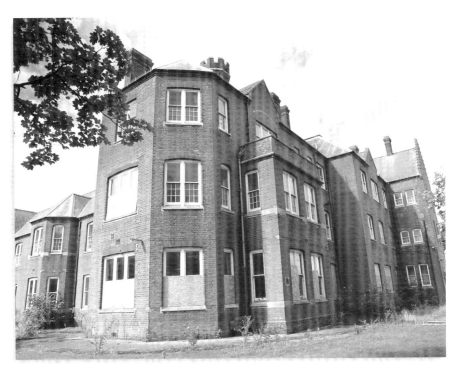

Male 6 (Frilsham) ward with Male 7 (Grazeley) above. (Bill Nicholls)

13

DERELICTION AND REDEVELOPMENT

....

A year or two later, Fair Mile enjoyed brief celebrity status when it was the film location for an episode of the popular *Midsomer Murders* television series, in an episode called 'The Silent Land'. The old asylum convincingly carried off the part of St Fidelis Hospital, a derelict tuberculosis sanatorium.

The hospital's closure left the community of Cholsey with a sense of loss; a kind of vacuum after 133 years of interaction; an old habit that had to be given up. There was real affection for the place, not so much for its echoing corridors, peeling paint and red-brick walls as for its sense of community and its mission of care. Would the new facility at Prospect Park, Reading, perform well? Would it uphold the Fair Mile traditions, even with many of the same personnel? Would 'Care in the Community' prove successful at the supervised accommodation units set up in Cholsey for vulnerable patients who, although no longer in need of acute care, had no other place to call home?

The most obvious question on Cholsey's collective mind concerned the future of the hospital's buildings and land, which were worth a king's ransom to any predatory developer: images of wrecking balls and a carpet of cheaply built, shoebox-sized homes stretching from the A329 to the Thames gave rise to many a worried conversation. Some imagined the place being turned into a conference centre, at a time when they were so commonplace that attending conferences had become more popular than working for a living. Thankfully, Cholsey – already in the habit of looking out for its best interests – was blessed with the good sense and initiative to organise a liaison committee to monitor events. After several years of high-level negotiations between local authorities, the NHS, developers, financiers and architects, a set of proposals was presented to the village in an exemplary manner. Architects John Thompson & Partners held several public meetings to tune into local concerns and views, organised workshops in which residents not only voiced their opinions but collaborated and used their local knowledge to develop ideas and policies and to identify issues – and every promise of information was fulfilled.

Whilst we may be entitled to a dash of cynicism over whether local concerns are ever actually taken into account in such situations, the plans that were subsequently made public were no discredit to either the architects or South Oxfordshire District Council (SODC). It was confirmed that the Victorian buildings enjoyed Grade II listed status and there was relief at the news that Marnock's elegant grounds were similarly protected. In fact, the South Oxfordshire Local Plan of 1997 had taken stock of Fair Mile's impending closure and made a number of explicit decisions affording protection from reckless exploitation.

Thompson's vision saw the hospital buildings transformed into modern, energy-efficient apartments and houses, with demolition largely confined to the unprepossessing twentieth-century wings, a number of dilapidated industrial build-ings, parts of the farm site and a few other impractical and architecturally low-grade structures. Locals would, however, have to tolerate the demolition of Rotherfield Ward (the much-loved 'Bungalow'), the Villa, Brightwell House, the hostels and the Super's house. Also on the agenda for removal was the complex of buildings occu-pied by the still-vigorous FMSSC. The Schuster was to be the largest single casualty. Notwithstanding its architectural award, it had not proved durable and was by now vandalised and in a sorry state.

Alongside the Victorian hospital, which would revert more or less to its 1904 layout, new houses and flats would be built to the north-east and south-west, mostly on land made available by demolition. The housing would include apartments of various sizes, social housing, live/work units for small businesses and some spa-cious dwellings with commanding views towards the Thames. Whilst new buildings hugged the north and south boundaries, the land between the old asylum and the river was to remain completely unspoilt; the cricket field would be reinstated and its pavilion refurbished; there would be meadows, footpaths and allotments, not to mention a number of eco-friendly proposals, including one to reopen the artesian wells[42].

Local reaction was favourable and discussion turned to such mundane consid-erations as access and parking, traffic calming and the profitable use of the former chapel and Recreation Hall. The FMSSC would have to vacate its clubhouse but much energy was expended on identifying a new home. Another significant con-sideration, much discussed from an early stage, was the careful integration of the new-style Fair Mile community into the village as a whole.

Developers Linden Homes and Thomas Homes became the new joint owners of a sad-looking piece of real estate, and security fencing went up in an attempt to deter the less kindly disposed class of visitor. Linden would attend to new-build construction, styling their offerings *Cholsey Meadows*, while Thomas Homes faced the daunting task of converting 312,000sq.ft (29,000sq.m) of draughty and dilapidated Victorian wards, offices and corridors into stylish and energy-efficient independent homes that were fully attuned to the age of the smartphone and rocketing energy prices. With an eye to continuity, they elected to retain the *Fair Mile* name and adopted a number of the original ward names to identify areas of housing.

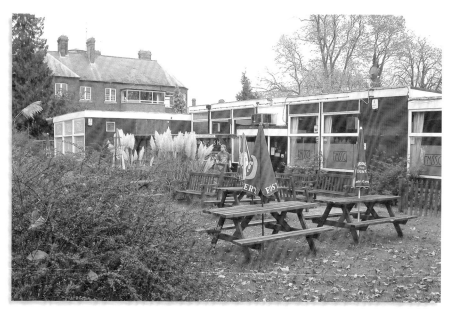

The FMSSC premises in 2010, just before they were demolished. The interior was more
capacious and comfortable than this view suggests. (Tony Rayner)

The recessionary hammer blows of 2008 then caused everyone, including the
planning authorities, to re-examine their financial calculations and mark time for
nearly two years before there was a reasonable expectation of sufficient buyers to
make it worth placing one brick on top of another.

The George Schuster Hospital was the first area scheduled for demolition, standing
as it did outside the main site; the bulldozers arrived in 2010 and properties were on
sale in 2011. Within the original grounds, the first impact was the shock announce-
ment that the FMSSC buildings would be the first to come down – at unexpectedly
short notice. This revelation created a justifiable storm of protest from FMSSC, which
had been led to expect adequate provision in the redundant chapel. Fortunately,
a nearby pub had recently ceased trading and assistance was provided to relocate
the club a couple of hundred metres up the road into the old-established Morning
Star, although not without significant reduction in the facilities it formerly boasted.
This interim measure proved successful enough that the club had embarked on purchasing the pub before Fair Mile's redevelopment had been completed.

After closure, and while the future of Fair Mile remained uncertain, an entirely
new class of visitor made its presence felt on the hospital site. Students of dereliction
with an interest in history in the raw found their way – not always entirely legally –
into the grounds and buildings, armed with curiosity and cameras. The fascinating
photographic records that resulted are readily found on the Internet. Photographs
of ruined workshops and broken-down interiors, long-abandoned bathrooms and
ghost-filled corridors are poignant reminders of better days and of a lost purpose.

Knowing that his research was supported by the developers, the author takes pleasure in recommending the work of Cholsey resident Bill Nicholls, who photographed the hospital extensively through the dereliction and redevelopment phases and published an illustrated blog at forgottenfairmile.blogspot.co.uk. Some of Bill's photographs are reproduced herein with his kind permission.

What's in a Name?

Early in the redevelopment process, SODC approached the village's liaison committee, soliciting help with road naming. The author, having the most obvious fund of information, was able to supply a hasty and highly provisional selection of names but requested a street plan and time to come up with a list that reflected the notable features and personalities in Fair Mile's history. Unaccountably, SODC claimed there was no time for lengthy deliberation and promptly closed the book on the matter. Thus it is that, years later, we find Villa Close on the site of South Lodge. Equally curious, though pleasing, was the discovery of Ruttle Close, named after Chris Ruttle who worked in the laundry in the post-war years. An alternative claimant might be his brother Albie, who delivered coal to the wards. As we have Chris's likeness, we will assume that he has the honour, no doubt sharing it with Joan Woodward, manageress of the laundry, who has her own road close by. Both were popular and they loved each other deeply. These lifelong partners would probably be amused – and also pleased – that Fair Mile has been remembered for its people.

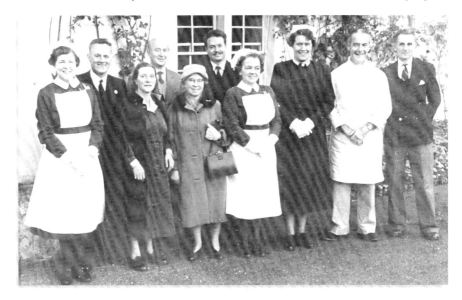

From left: Sister Morfydd Jones; 'Taff' Jones; Lilian Talbot; Leslie Talbot; Alice 'Tot' Gibbons (sister of Mrs Talbot); unknown; Edith Meatyard; Matron Smythe; Harry Beasley (chef); George Hedges (electrician). (Spackman collection)

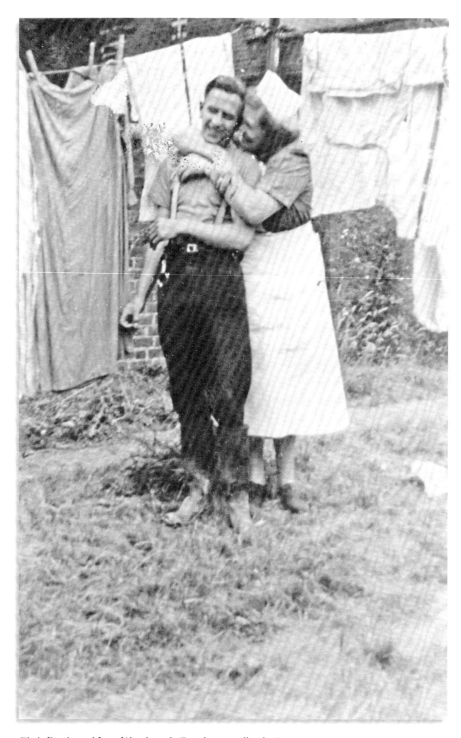

Chris Ruttle and Joan Woodward. (Spackman collection)

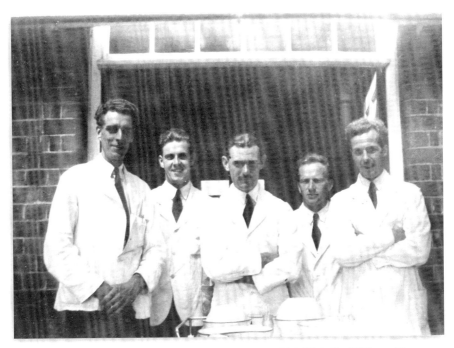

Male nursing staff in about 1948. From left: Lem White; Dick Nicholls; Alf Reynolds; possibly Jock Oliver; Peter Vick. (Bill Nicholls)

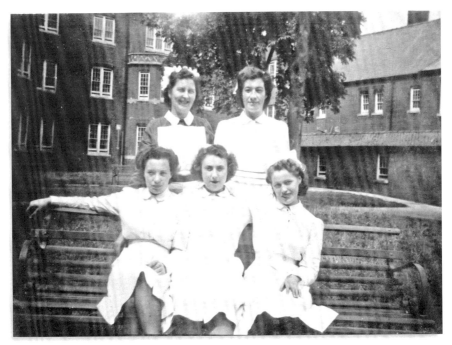

Nurses in the female airing court in about 1950. Rear left is Molly Brady; May Lehaney rear right. Carmel Clancy front left. (Bill Nicholls)

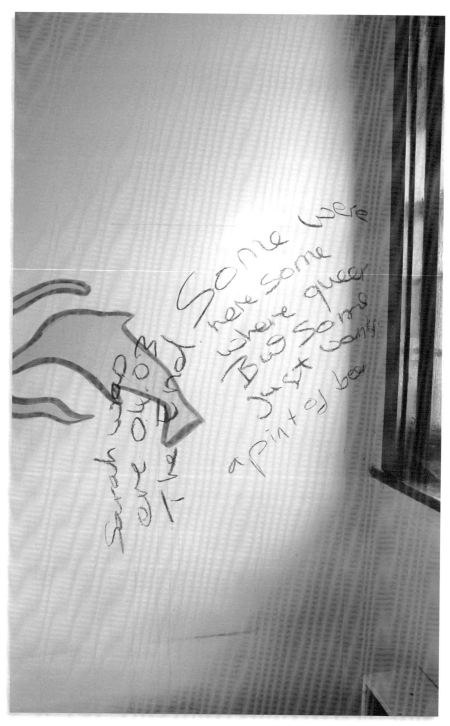

A patient's graffito says it all. (Bill Nicholls)

ACKNOWLEDGEMENTS, SOURCES AND REFERENCES

I am deeply grateful to the many people who have provided material for this book. I have done what was possible to crosscheck information supplied in good faith but, inevitably, there will be mistakes and omissions for which I can only apologise. Any corrections reaching my attention will be incorporated into the continuing research on this fascinating establishment.

It has proven quite impossible to mention everyone whose name has come my way in the course of research. Every single Fair Mile patient and employee is important to this account and I regret that space has not allowed everyone's story to be told.

For many forms of involvement, thanks are due to:

The National Archives via the Internet; Lionel Baldwin; David Beasley; Hilda Behan; Charles Bosher of Boshers (Cholsey) Ltd; Renee Brewerton; Kitty Brown; Peter and Maureen Caton; Chris Chapman; Valerie Collett; Gladys Curtis; Fran De Condé; Fred Derrick; the late Stuart Dewey; Judy Dewey; Sheila Drinkall; Mary Dyson; Sylvia Farney; Gladys Fox; Pat Green; the late Jeannine Grigoriwicz; Lena Haynes; Bill Holliday; Paul Holmes; Epsom & Ewell History Explorer www.epsomandewellhistoryexplorer.org.uk; Joan Hudson; Bill Lane; John Lias; Peter Lines; Wilf, Rosie and Ron Marshall; John and Jeanne Money; Caro Muir; Bill Nicholls; Rose Noorduijn; Isobel Perry; Nigel Peterson; Revd Andrew Petit; Frank and Tina Plazas; Ken and Conchita Polley; the late Gwilym Pryce; Miriam Pryce; Tony Rayner; Roland Raynor; Michael Reynolds; Annie Rickard; Charles and Lynn Rigby; Angela Rowlands; Linda Saunders; Pam Seymour; June Smith; Peter Smithers; Tony Spackman; Mark Stevens of the Berkshire Record Office; the late John Talbot; the late Lilian Talbot; David Talbot; Mildred Taylor; Dr John Beckerson and John Horne of the National Gas Museum, Leicester; Sue Clarke of the Winterbourne Therapeutic Community, Reading; Vera Wheeler; Lesley Whittaker, Rod and June Wilkins; Audrey Woodage; Mary Woollard; Momena and Robert Wright; Brian Wyatt; Carolyn Wyatt; the late Gerald 'Jed' Wyatt; Renato and Angela Zito.

I would also like to thank Cholsey 1000 Plus for facilitating two showings of *Fair Mile's Forgotten Faces*, the exhibition that led to this book, and for their enduring support of local historical research.

Many thanks to Chris Brotherton of Thomas Homes, for tours of the redevelopment site, information and drawings adapted for use in this book.

Special thanks to Diana M. DeLuca PhD for her contribution relating to her mother, the late Mary Fairbairn Macintyre. Further information has been drawn from Mary's fascinating book, *Nursing at The Fairmile Mental Hospital, Cholsey 1935–1939*, which chronicles her training period at the Berkshire Mental Hospital and was published by the Berkshire Medical Heritage Centre, Royal Berkshire Hospital, Reading, in 2013.

Great credit must also go to Judy and the late Stuart Dewey, authors of *Change at Cholsey – Again!* (Pie Powder Press, 2001), not only for facts about Fair Mile but also for their work in encouraging research into Cholsey's past.

Cholsey historian Barrie Charles examines a number of events associated with the asylum's early years in *Crime and Calamity in Cholsey* (Lulu.com, 2013).

Extensive amounts of information, distributed throughout this work, have also been drawn from the Berkshire Record Office, Reading, principally:

- Visitors' minutes D/H 10/A1/1
- General Statement book D/H 10/A4/1
- Hine's 1898 specifications for extensions D/H 10/B1/3
- Superintendent's journals D/H 10/A4/1 to -8
- Chaplain's Journal D/H 10/E/1/1 to -15
- Annual reports of the Commissioners D/H 10/A2/1; D/H 10/A2/2;
- Annual Reports of the Medical Superintendent and principal officers Q/AL 12

Although not used as a source, Mark Stevens' *Life in the Victorian Asylum* (Pen & Sword, 2014) contains much supplementary information based on the Fair Mile archives.

Many evocative photographs of the dereliction and redevelopment periods can be found on these and other websites:

forgottenfairmile.blogspot.co.uk
www.derelictplaces.co.uk/main/showthread.php?t=24331#.U7PPjEDpf6I
www.whateversleft.co.uk/asylums/fairmile-hospital-berkshire

NOTES

1   The county line between Oxfordshire and Berkshire was changed in 1974, leaving Fair Mile a few miles inside Oxfordshire's southern border.

2   Accounts of the land area vary according to source but a more recent figure of 97 acres would include the later Schuster Hospital.

3   Invariably known to Cholsey residents as Ferry Lane, while official records sometimes consider this to be an extension of Papist Way.

4   The first report of the Committee of Visitors described it as 'a modification of early English'.

5   It has been said that, in addition to exotic specimens that still survive, there was at least one example of every native British tree.

6   Later revealed to be Berkshire residents.

7   Literally, 'one holding a place'. We nowadays use only locum.

8   An early duplicating machine by Hungarian-born David Gestetner but nevertheless a British invention.

9   This was a system for monitoring staff vigilance, especially at night, when the attendant was expected to 'punch a clock' every half hour.

10   Some sources, including the National Archives, quote the date of his departure as 1946 but 1944 has been found in the archives, with indication that it was late in the year. He had certainly vacated by July 1945.

11   The Clerk of Works was initially needed to oversee the construction of the new asylum but Superintendent Gilland begged leave from Mansfield, Price & Co., the building contractors, to retain his services to attend to a steady stream of maintenance, repair and improvement demands.

12   Mr Petrocokino's distinctive name has been noticed as late as 1924, suggesting yeoman service.

13   The Berkshire Record Office states that inspections took place twice a year but the available commissioners' reports from 1923 are certainly annual.

14   Gas lighting had a protracted development history; some Chinese were burning natural gas for lighting in the fourth century.

15   It is unlikely that the 1910 purchase of engine and dynamo had been finalised.

16   Other contenders included the equally famous Edison Swan, British Thomson Houston Co. and Siemens Bros., whose even more economical 'Wotan' lamps were later purchased.

17   Compare this with a modern 60W lamp, which emits about 65 candlepower.

18   Yeast was a major product of the Distillers Company Ltd.

19   James Morrison (1789–1857) was a fabulously rich, self-made businessman and Member of Parliament. His descendants were notable landowners for many years.

20   A calming therapy in which patients would spend hours or sometimes days suspended in warm water that was continuously replenished.

21   The gardens later became a tennis court, which can be seen in some of the aerial photographs.

22 Also visible in the 1870 engraving in Chapter 1.

23 Journals of around 1935 make passing references to 'the old villa', which still existed, but no clear idea of what this might have been has come to light, unless it was the original superintendent's house.

24 The Commissioner's report of 1935 states explicitly that the house was for female staff working in the Villa but first-hand witnesses are sure it was for the matron. Arrangements changed from about 1955 and the matron had an apartment above the administration block in the 1960s.

25 Not one of the classifications under the Idiots Act of 1886 but nevertheless an official term.

26 The term 'inmate', although tempting, was rarely used.

27 'Soft' is a relative term; this was probably Bronco, also known as 'rough and shiny'.

28 As the Bungalow (see Chapter 4) did not exist at this time, this would be one of the infirmary wards.

29 These statements are mysterious, since both Female 8 and Male 8 already had verandahs large enough to be seen on maps by 1936.

30 These men were fortunate to have Male 4 to themselves and, to all intents and purposes, their own staff.

31 Sharp-eyed readers will notice that this does not agree with other figures drawn from the same year's report.

32 Registered Mental Nurse.

33 Pictured in Chapter 3.

34 Some official records as early as 1911 use 'nurse', while former staff members claim that 'attendant' was current well into the 1930s.

35 These laboured under the lengthy title of Regulations and Orders for the Management and Conduct of those engaged in the Service of the Berkshire Asylum Wallingford (see also Chapter 6).

36 Women took to this title more readily than men, who apparently thought of themselves as 'attendants' for years afterwards.

37 Leslie Talbot held this position at the time.

38 This was almost certainly Jack Croxford.

39 More likely, no more could be found to put up with the hours and conditions.

40 A salacious story related in detail in Barrie Charles' *Crime and Calamity in Cholsey*.

41 A loose term for which the author craves indulgence; the skill and dedication of modern psychiatric care staff is not in question but the emergence of sophisticated drugs was instrumental in a steady reduction in patient numbers that finally did away with the asylum in its familiar form.

42 This one at least did not make it past the planning authorities but perhaps a future generation will one day rediscover the delights of unadulterated drinking water.

INDEX
(PEOPLE)

....

See general index for organisations and companies.

Entries quoting only an initial are male. Married women are indexed by their maiden names but either surname may appear in the text or captions.

Bold type denotes an illustration.

INDEX
(GENERAL)

....

Bold type denotes an illustration

Also from The History Press

BACK TO
SCHOOL

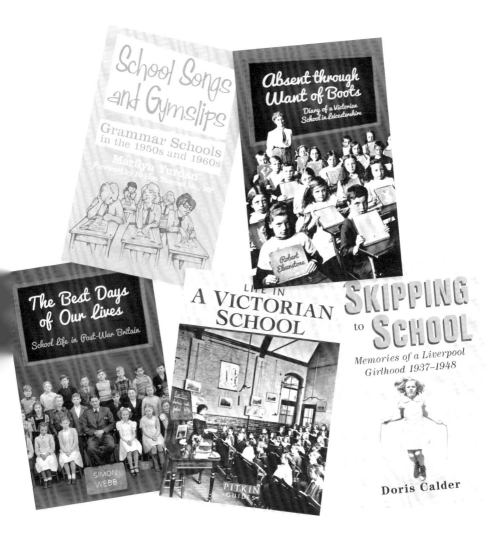

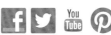

The History Press

Also from The History Press

Victorian Villains

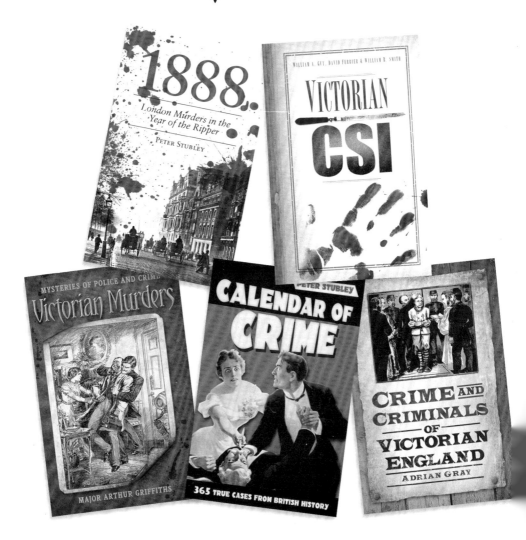